KETOGENIC DIET FOR WOMEN AFTER 50

The Healthiest Lifestyle For Women Over 50 to Lose Weight, Reverse Disease and Feel Younger. Bonus: 7 Simple Exercises and a 30-Day Meal Plan

Suzanne Busy

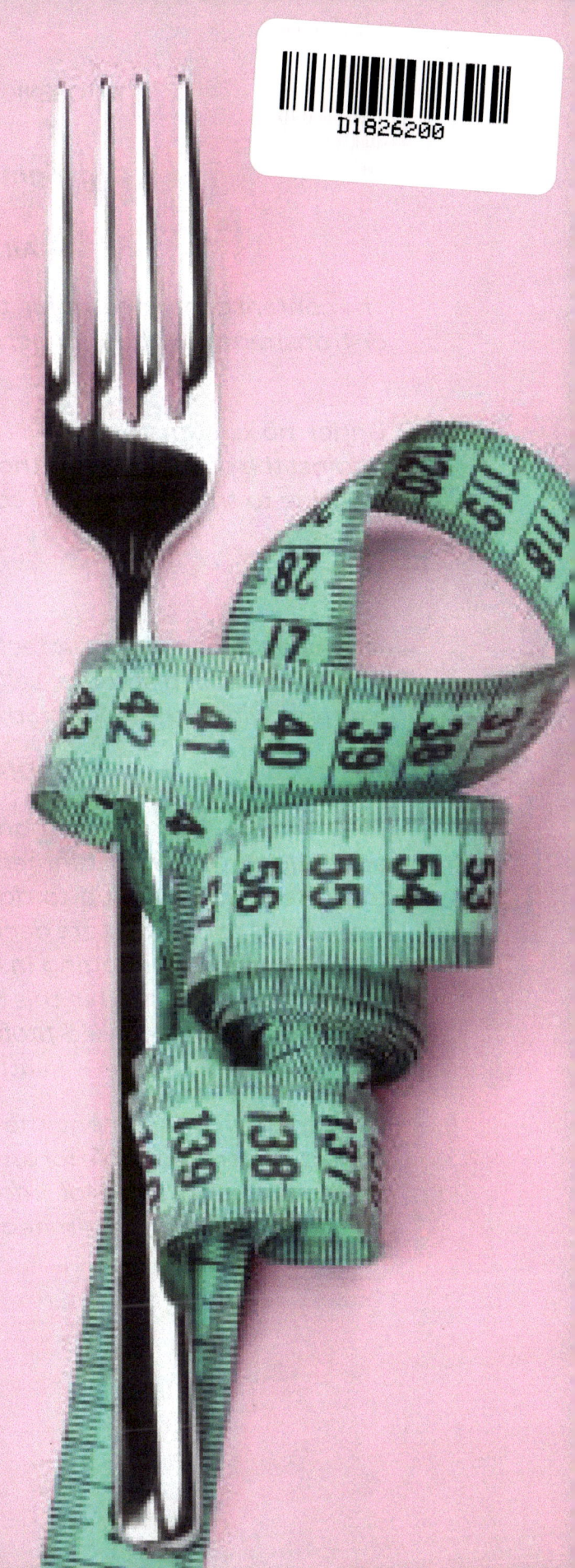

Disclaimer Notice:

2

Please note the information contained within this document is for educational and entertainment purposes only. All effort has been executed to present accurate, up to date, and reliable, complete information. No warranties of any kind are declared or implied. Readers acknowledge that the author is not engaging in the rendering of legal, financial, medical or profes The content within this book has been derived from various sources. Please consult a licensed professional before attempting any techniques outlined in this book.

By reading this document, the reader agrees that under no circumstances is the author responsible for any losses, direct or indirect, which are incurred as a result of the use of information contained within this document, including, but not limited to, - errors, omissions, or inaccuracies.

Table of Content

3

4

Suzanne Busy

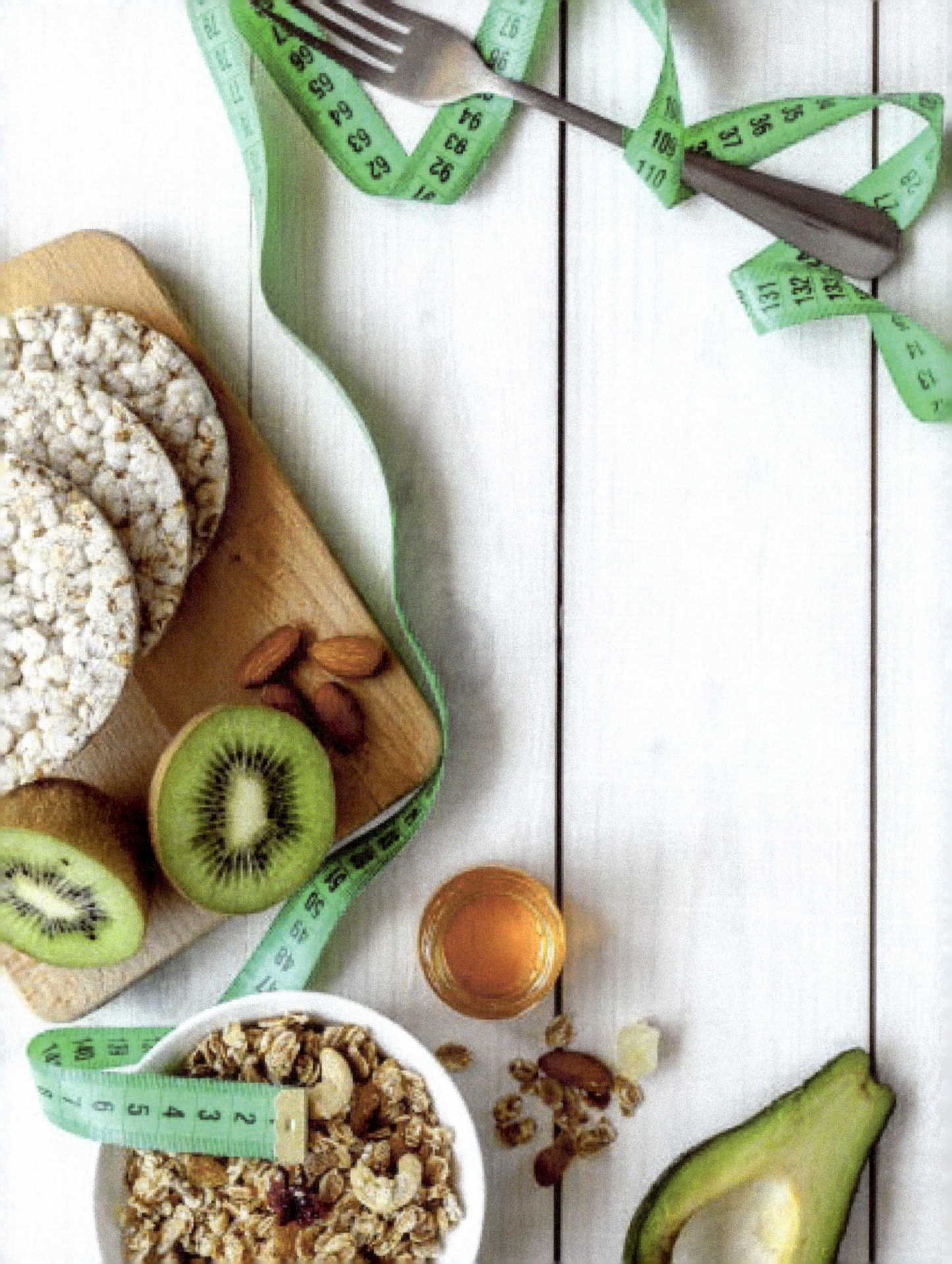

Introduction

The idea behind most diets remains the same. One needs to reduce the amount of carbs intake in a day, and the weight should fall. The problem is that most diets require you to stop eating or skip meals to bring the carb level down.

Indeed, the idea of losing weight is appealing. It is a motivator that pushes us to stop eating and force our body to start converting stored fats into fuel to burn. Sounds good, but the hunger that comes in is a killer.

The catch behind cutting down on carbs is simple; it makes your body run low on glucose. When that happens, the state of ketosis is in effect. That is where ketones come to the rescue as your body's natural fuel backup. Here's a little fact: we only ever enter into the state of ketosis if we starve ourselves for a few days, not just overnight or by skipping a meal. That, then, is quite a challenging prospect.

It goes without saying that for a weight loss solution, Keto stands up as a perfect contender. No need to give up eating, but you can enjoy delicious dishes while you are losing your weight through easy steps that otherwise would require you to starve to near death. Additionally, most of these recipes are exceptionally easy to cook, and most of them taste equally delicious.

The ketogenic diet is trendy, and for an excellent reason. It truly

7

teaches healthy eating without forcing anyone into a risk. The success rate of Keto is relatively high. While there are no specific numbers to suggest the exact rate, it is only fair to state that those who have the will to change their lifestyle and are okay adjusting to new eating habits, almost every one of them will make it through as a success story.

As you grow in age, the body's natural fat-burning ability reduces. When that happens, your body stops receiving a healthy dose of nutrients properly, which is why you will develop diseases and ailments. With the keto diet, you are pushing the body into ketosis and bypassing the need to worry about your body's ability to burn fat. Once in ketosis, your body will now burn fat forcefully for survival.

8

It is also essential to highlight that as we get older, we start losing more than just the ability to burn fat. During this phase of our life, once we hit around 50 years of age, we come across various obstacles, some chronic in nature, which transpire only because our body is no longer able to function at rates like it did when we were young. Ketogenic diets help us regain that edge and feel energized from within. It is, therefore, a no-brainer for women above 50 who have spent ages trying to search for a healthy lifestyle choice of diet. With such a high success rate, there is no harm in trying, right?

All in all, the keto diet is shaping up to be quite a promising candidate for older adults. Not only will this diet allow us to lead a healthier lifestyle, but it will also curb our ailments and ensure high energy around the clock.

Keto has been producing results that have attracted the top minds and researchers for a reasonably long time. With the unique nature of this lifestyle of eating, the results have been somewhat encouraging.

9

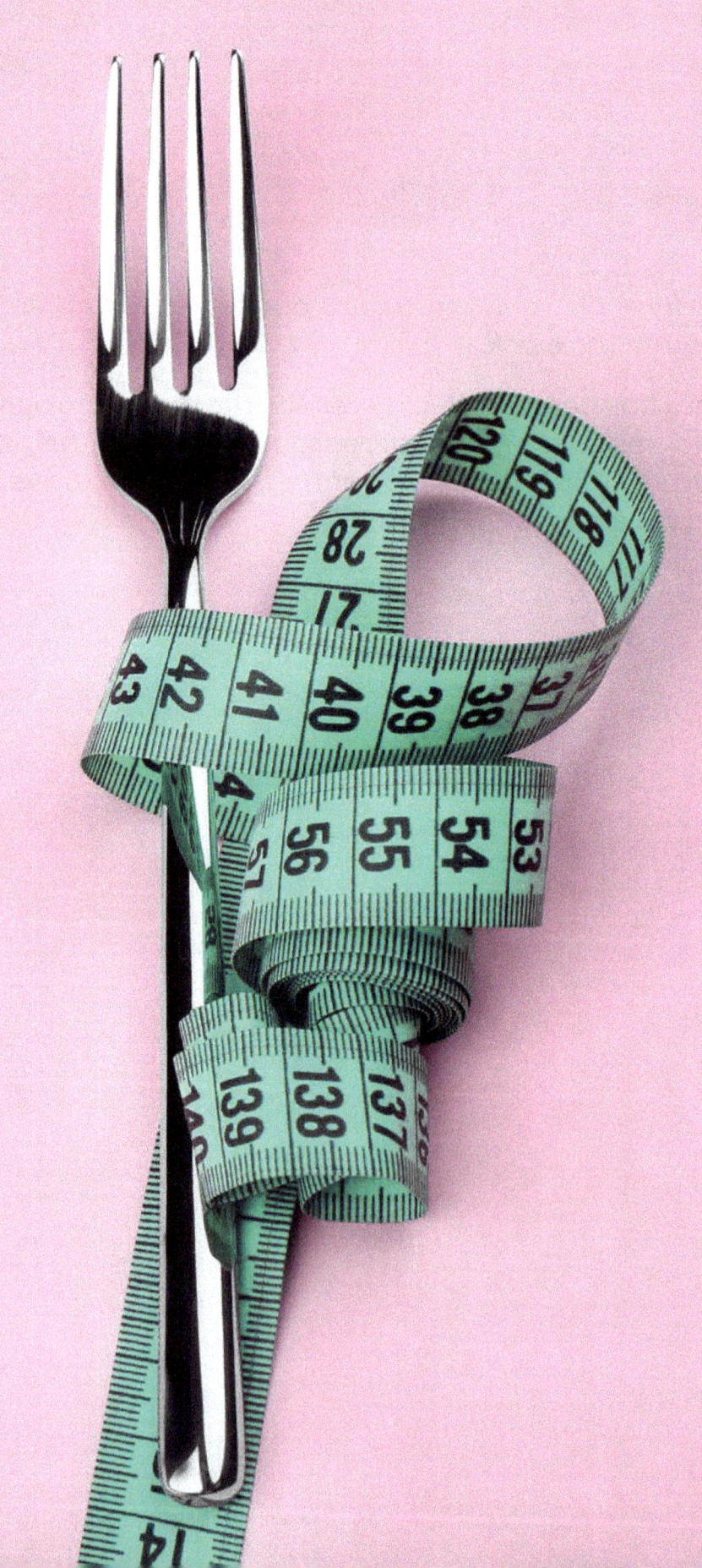

Chapter 01

What Ketogenic Diet Is and the Why of Keto

A diet that results in the production of ketone bodies by the liver is called a ketogenic diet; it causes your system to use fat instead of carbohydrates for energy. Limit your carbohydrate intake to a low level, causing some reactions. However, it is not a high protein diet. It involves moderate protein, low carbohydrate intake, and high fat intake. The exact percentage of macronutrients varies according to your needs. Fats make up 75% of the calories you eat, making them a key component of your diet, protein makes up 30% of the calories you eat, and carbohydrates 10%.

Your system generally works with a mixture of proteins, carbohydrates, and fats. This diet eliminates carbohydrates, which causes the system's reserves to be depleted and the body to find an alternative source of energy.

11

Insufficient free fatty acid disintegration releases as by-product ketone bodies. The energy supplied is fat obtained without carbohydrates, which is used by organs such as the brain. As a consequence of the rapid manufacturing of ketone bodies, which makes them accumulate in the blood, ketosis develops. The manufacture and use of glucose in your system are also reduced; the protein used for power is also reduced.

The levels of glucagon and glucose are affected by ketogenic diets. Insulin transforms glucose into glycogen that is recycled as fat, while glucagon transforms glycogen into glucose to provide your system with power. Carbs removal from the diet improves the levels of glucagon and decreases levels of insulin. This, in the end, causes the liberation of an increased number of FFA and their decomposition in the liver that results in the manufacturing of ketone bodies and induces the ketosis state.

In a way, the diet is identical to starvation, with the distinction being that there is food intake in one. The metabolic impacts that come about and the adjustments experienced in starvation are approximately the same as those experienced during the diet. There has been an extensive study of the reaction to complete hunger, probably more so than the diet on its own. That's why the vast bulk of the information described is derived from the analyses of fasting individuals. There are few exceptions, but the diet's metabolic impacts are similar to those that occur during starvation. The reactions in ketosis as a result of carb restriction are the same as the reactions seen with starvation. In this regard, protein and fat amounts are not that important.

There is no one-size-fits-all when it comes to how much of your total calorie requirement you should derive from carbs. Some nutritionists advise people to keep it in the low end, which is five percent, but it is not necessarily good advice as the exact amount depends on your system. To get the right amount for you will have to rely on the trial and error method. Select a percentage and see how it feels for you; if you don't like the results, you can adjust accordingly. With fats and protein, just like in carbs, there is no exact amount for

12

everyone. It all depends on you, but seventy-five percent is a good place to start off.

There is no space to "cheat" your diet here. You should follow it completely as even one meal that does not follow its rules can slow down your advancement for about a week as your body is withdrawn from ketosis. Always make sure you've eaten enough so that you will not be tempted to have a snack that could ruin all you've been working for.

As we age, we naturally lose energy. While it might have previously been easy to work a full-time job and then go partying through all hours of the night, as we get older, we find that just doing what we have to do gets exhausting. But, there are ways we can increase our energy. By changing your diet, you will find that you have the capabilities to not only do more but feel better while you do it. You have most likely heard the phrase "you are what you eat" your entire life. While this phrase may not be literal, what you eat does become the fuel for your cells, which then affects how you can live. If you give your body poor quality fuel, you will find your energy and health plummet. On the other hand, if you give your body healthy and high-quality fuel, you will increase your energy, well-being, and overall quality of life.

13

When on a standard Western diet, also frequently referred to as the Standard American Diet (SAD), people consume large quantities of carbs and highly processed additives. After we eat these carbs, whether it is ice cream and cookies or a bowl of pasta and French *bread, these carbs are broken down into glucose by the body. This glucose is pure sugar, which is being fed to our cells as fuel.*

When your body uses glucose as the fuel, you get a temporary sugar-high, just like a child who gets a burst of energy after eating an ice cream cone. However, when this happens, insulin must be released by your pancreas in an attempt to manage the high blood sugar levels.

Sadly, this process, which should go smoothly in healthy individuals, frequently becomes impeded due to a variety of health conditions or old age. For instance, insulin resistance and reduced insulin sensitivity frequently can make it difficult for the insulin response to manage blood sugar, frequently leading to diabetes.

14 *When insulin is unable to manage our blood sugar in a healthy way, then we experience two extremes. After all, for every action, there is an equal and opposite reaction. The first extreme you experience is the sugar high, and while this may give you a temporary surge of energy, it is frantic and unhealthy energy, one of which is only short-lasting.*

After your short energy comes to the shock of sugar, just as the sugar rush causes extreme nervousness and energy, the sugar crash causes extreme fatigue, drowsiness, and headaches. Even people with a healthy insulin response experience this sugar high and crash, and it is only worsened as people age or develop insulin-related disorders.

While carbohydrates create glucose, a sugar, as a fuel source, the ketogenic diet greatly limits your carbohydrate intake. Because of this, instead of relying on quick sugar highs for energy, your body will rely on healthier and slower burning fuel sources. Fat and protein burn more slowly and without either a high or a crash, allowing your body to maintain a healthy and sustained energy level.

Not only will you have the longer burning fuel of fat and protein, but your body will also produce ketone bodies for fuel once you have adapted to the diet and reached the stage of ketosis. When this happens, the ketones will help fuel your body whenever you need an added boost of energy, ensuring that you have fewer energy crashes. No longer will you have to push through those dreaded afternoon slumps, Mondays will become easier, and you will find yourself drinking less caffeine. Between fat, protein, and ketones, you will be providing your body and cells with the best fuel sources they could hope for, allowing you to enjoy the all-day energy you have desired.

15

MITOCHONDRIAL BENEFITS

The mitochondrial cells, which are the cells that have the capability of using any of the fuel sources of energy, are incredibly powerful. The mitochondria within these cells are frequently referred to as the "powerhouse of the cell." The reason they are so powerful is that they produce ninety percent of the energy humans need to survive.

When we breathe the mitochondria, use a process known as oxidative phosphorylation to combine oxygen and the fuel we have eaten to create ATP energy. But, when there is a malfunction in the mitochondria, they are unable to fully produce the amount of ATP energy re requiring, resulting in damaged cells, tissues, and even organs.

These mitochondrial disorders can be inherited genetically or caused by various environmental factors. Thankfully, you can improve your mitochondrial and overall health by changing the fuel you feed your cells. By giving them higher quality fats, proteins, and ketones rather than low-quality glucose, you can impact the health of your entire body, as the mitochondrial cells make up such a large portion of your body.

16

Promising research has found that the ketogenic diet can increase the rate of energy synthesis by mitochondrial cells, thereby reducing or preventing the energy deficiencies that go hand-in-hand with mitochondrial disorders. Not only that, but the ketogenic diet can also increase the number of mitochondrial cells found within the human body, increasing the energy even further.

BEAUTIFUL HEALTHY SKIN AND HAIR

We all want to have beautiful skin and hair. But, as we age, they often lose their shine, become rough and course, and we may struggle with hair loss or skin rashes. When a person first begins the ketogenic diet, they may experience adverse side effects with their hair or skin, but this is due to the body's natural adjustment period. After you have been on the ketogenic diet for a few weeks or months, you should notice that your hair and skin begin to not only go back to normal but that they exceed their previous health.

This is largely due to overall body health, allowing your skin and hair to become the best version of themselves, but it is also due to providing them better fuel. The cells within your hair and skin require fuel just like all your other cells, but frequently, these cells are not given enough healthy fat. This reduction in fat causes brittle hair that has lost its shine and dry, itchy skin. But, if you provide these cells with healthy fats from avocados, olives, nuts, seeds, and fish, then you will find that they gain the luxurious health you have longed for.

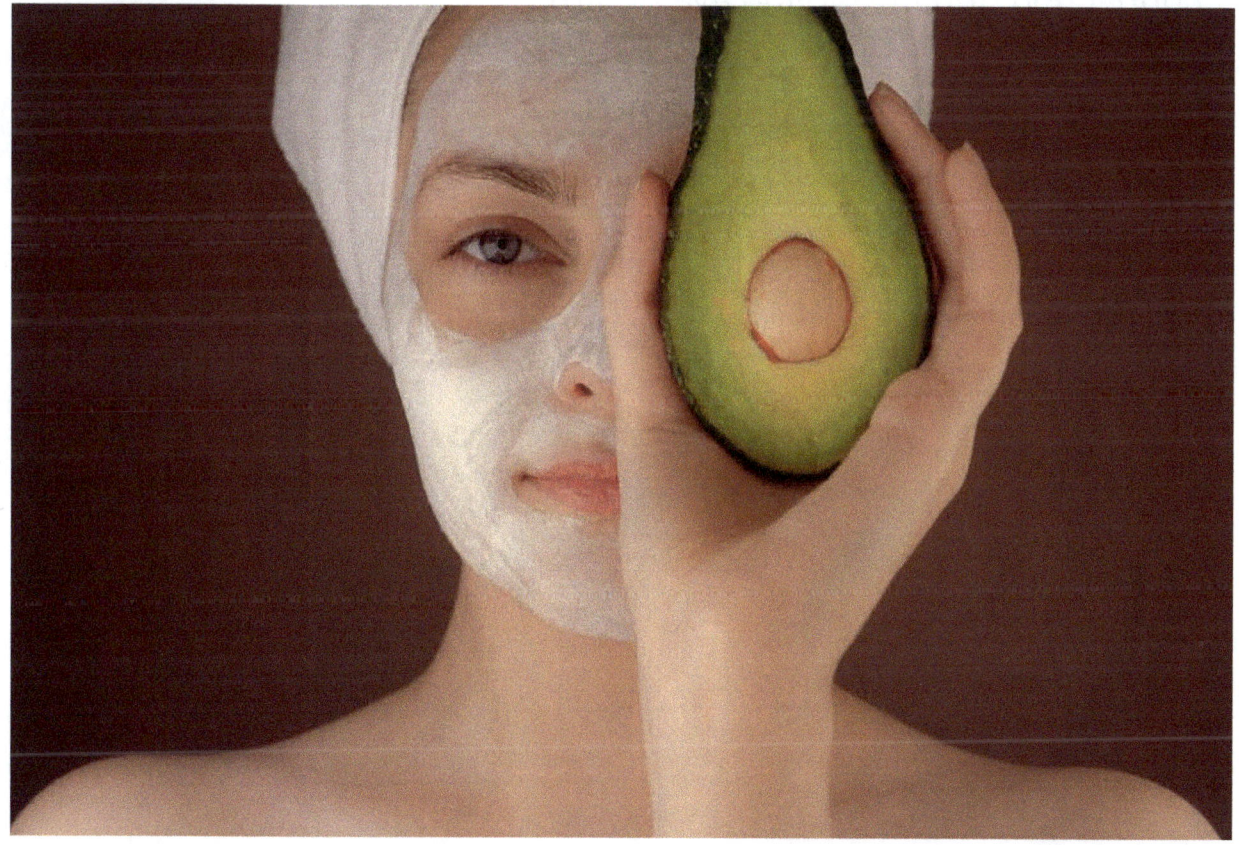

17

BOOST EYE HEALTH

As we age, our eye health degenerates. Sometimes, this reveals itself simply with the vision becoming poorer and blurrier, but other times, it causes glaucoma to develop. This progressive condition causes damage to the cells that communicate visual information between the eyes and brain. What many people may not know is that if you have diabetes or a family history of diabetes, then you are at a higher risk of developing glaucoma. Thankfully, a study found that maintaining a ketogenic diet helps to protect these cells, allowing the eyes and brain to retain their communication connection and preserving eye health.

18

Chapter 02

Macronutrients and Ketogenic

Unfortunately, one of the main aspects that you will not be able to eat whatever you want when you are following a keto diet. However, like many diets, you will have a wide array of options to choose from. You can find alternatives that you can enjoy and avoid a high carbohydrate diet. The essence of the keto diet is to get your body into ketosis, and all you need to do is to reduce your carbohydrate intake. Carbohydrates are not only the junk foods that you love but also some other healthier foods that you enjoy.

THE MACROS I SHOULD AIM FOR ON THE KETO DIET AFTER 50

Macro is a term that is coined from macronutrients, which include protein, fats, and carbohydrates, which makes up the composition of macronutrients required by the body. You can easily find this information listed on the nutritional facts panel of most foods, and you can use counting apps or calculators to calculate your macros. Gram for gram, the macronutrients are critical in the total calorie count that you will consume per day. One gram of carbohydrate will provide four calories; one gram of protein provides four calories, while one gram of fat will give you nine calories. Alcohol is also considered a macronutrient, and it gives seven calories per gram, although it has no nutritional value to the body.

When you follow your macro diet, you will go beyond counting calories, and you will focus more on macros. Depending on your

19

health objectives, you can adjust the ratios of the macronutrients that you consume to help you build muscle, lose weight, or enter a maintenance mode. If you follow a ketogenic diet, you will pay attention to net carbohydrates as part of the macros because it will determine how many useful carbohydrates you will consume per meal.

The macronutrients mustn't be confused with micronutrients, which are the key vitamins and minerals in the body. The micronutrients are required in small quantities, and they are essential in doing everything from regulating hormones to boosting brain performance. Macros are also different from the macrobiotic diet, which has principles drawn from Zen Buddhism.

KETO DIET MACROS BETWEEN MEN AND WOMEN AFTER 50

Macros zero in on the composition of your daily calories so that you can alter each to give you the best health that you want. If you have 70% calories in carbs, then you will feel different, unlike when you have 70% calories from fats. Men and women after 50 have to understand their macros so that they can adjust them according to their health and energy needs. With tracking, you can understand the source of the imbalance and make changes that will promote better growth and development of new cells.

Many people on a ketogenic diet will make the mistake of counting calories alone. This will not give them meaningful results because you will not know the balance of your energy source. If you want a more productive approach, you should monitor your macronutrients because it will tell you a more decent and better approach that you can use to achieve your health goals. Besides, when you follow the quality of your macros, you can potentially increase your fat-burning abilities and have a lean body.

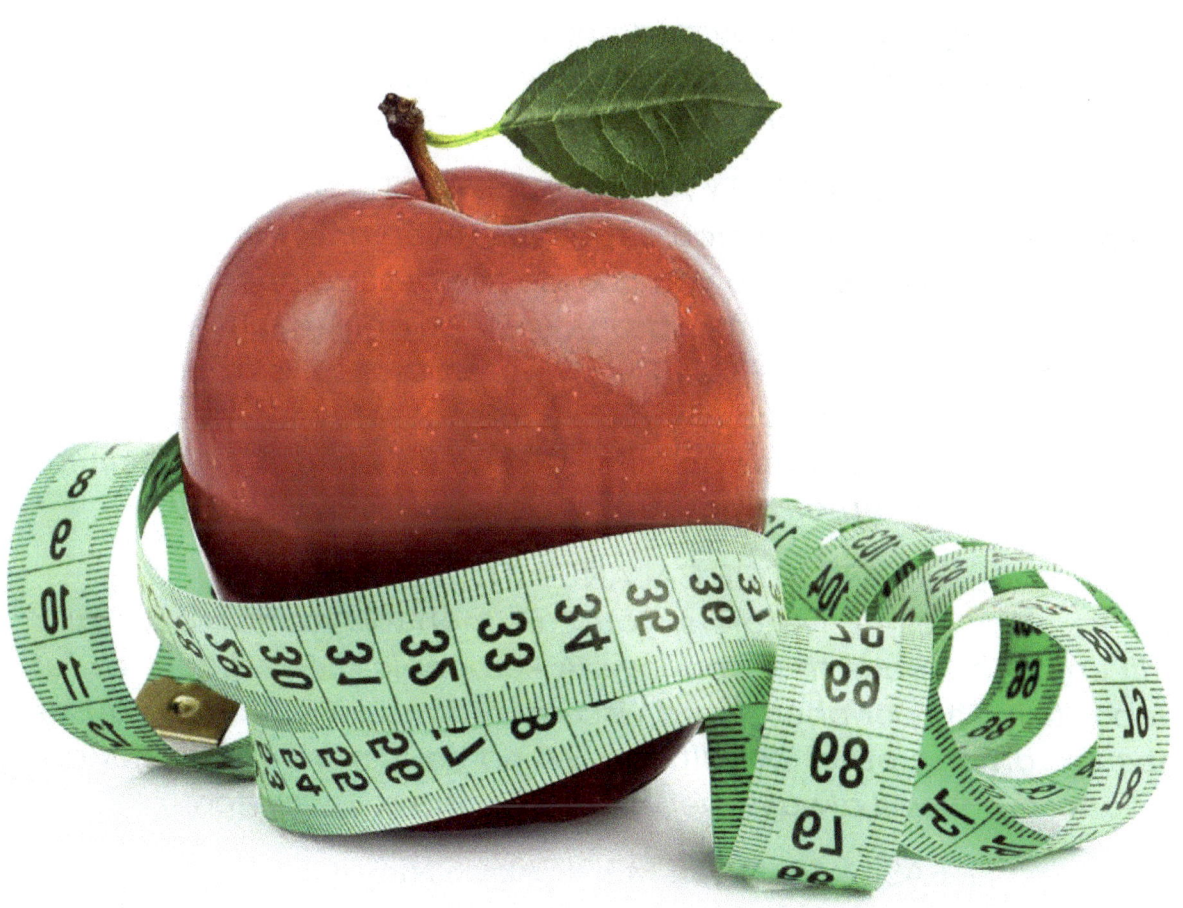

21

HOW CALORIES RESTRICTION SLOWS DOWN AGING

For anyone who has never tracked their calories and learned the quality ratio of protein, fat, and carbohydrates that are effective for their body, it can be unusual. When you monitor your calories for a few days, you will know what your body needs and what you can do to enhance your health. You need a diet that will give you adequate energy throughout the day and boost cellular regeneration. There are reasons why the restriction of calories will slow down the aging process. Some of the benefits of calorie restriction include:

FLEXIBILITY AND CUSTOMIZATION

There is no one size fits all macros because everyone has their health objectives. However, when you choose the best calorie intake that will put your health goals forward, you will be able to make the right decision and reduce the cellular aging process. It is important to understand that cells age when they are not rejuvenated properly. When you restrict calories and choose one which improves cellular division, you will remain youthful.

22

HAVE MORE BALANCE IN YOUR DIET

Unlike other restrictive diets, you can monitor your calories and still enjoy the foods that you love. A ketogenic diet will reduce fat deposits in the peripheral and visceral organs, which often causes obesity, among other conditions. When your macronutrients are balanced, you will always feel energized and rejuvenated.

EASILY MANAGE MEDICAL CONDITIONS

Some studies indicate that managing your calorie intake is essential in building a better feeling and rejuvenation. Studies indicate that the macronutrients will help you manage conditions such as diabetes, polycystic ovary syndrome, and certain cancers. You must consult your physician before cutting down your calories.

HOW AGING AFFECTS YOUR NUTRITIONAL NEEDS

Nutrition is vital in maintaining a healthy biological system. You can lead a happy and fulfilling life when you choose the right nutrition. However, it is imperative to understand that nutrition changes with age, and if you are suffering from nutritional deficiencies, then it will bring harmful outcomes. In the initial years of childhood, the little bodies will require essential nutrients to enable them to grow and develop quickly, both physically and mentally. The food should provide high energy as well as nourishing capabilities that can enhance the cognitive abilities of the child. It is also important to note that the child is learning new foods and developing their taste, which will shape their eating habits in the future. Therefore, the kids should be encouraged to consume a wide array of foods to help them get all the essential nutrients. The key nutrient includes proteins necessary for growth, Vitamin D to help in the growth of strong bones. Along with other vital nutrients such as vitamin A are vital in boosting the immune system, while zinc and iron are essential in boosting the mental abilities of the kids.

23

During adolescence, 13-19 years, the body is going around significant changes emotionally and physically because of puberty. Moreover, they are maturing now, and the growth of bones and muscles occurs during this phase. For this reason, you will require a diet that is rich in calcium, hence the importance of milk products. Iron is also an important component, and it can be obtained from meat, chicken, kidney beans, and spinach. During the teenage years, the body requires vital nutrients. Although many kids will want to switch to sugary foods and drinks, you should always encourage them to eat healthy foods because it will impact their life later.

Adulthood: 20 to 50 years, presents a myriad of challenges, and this is a time where you are required to maintain a healthy balance in the foods that you consume. The body cells are degenerating faster than they are being replaced hence the need to switch to a healthier diet and always consider your medical conditions. You should get enough nutrition of proteins, carbohydrates, and vitamins, as well as micronutrients. You must focus on a diet that will help you feel great without disturbing your body in terms of weight and emotional aspects. You need the energy to carry out your activities hence the need to balance your diet effectively.

24

Old age occurs when you are over 50 years, the body will need more vitamins, minerals, and proteins to help in building the cellular structure as well as maintain a good balance emotionally. The body's ability to absorb certain nutrients diminishes as you go past 50 years, and it is therefore important that you choose a diet that will replenish your nutrients regularly. If you are taking a diet that does not have all the essential minerals and vitamins, then you should consider adding supplements to your diet. You should look at your body needs by monitoring the calories and macros because this will give you the best emotional and body balance.

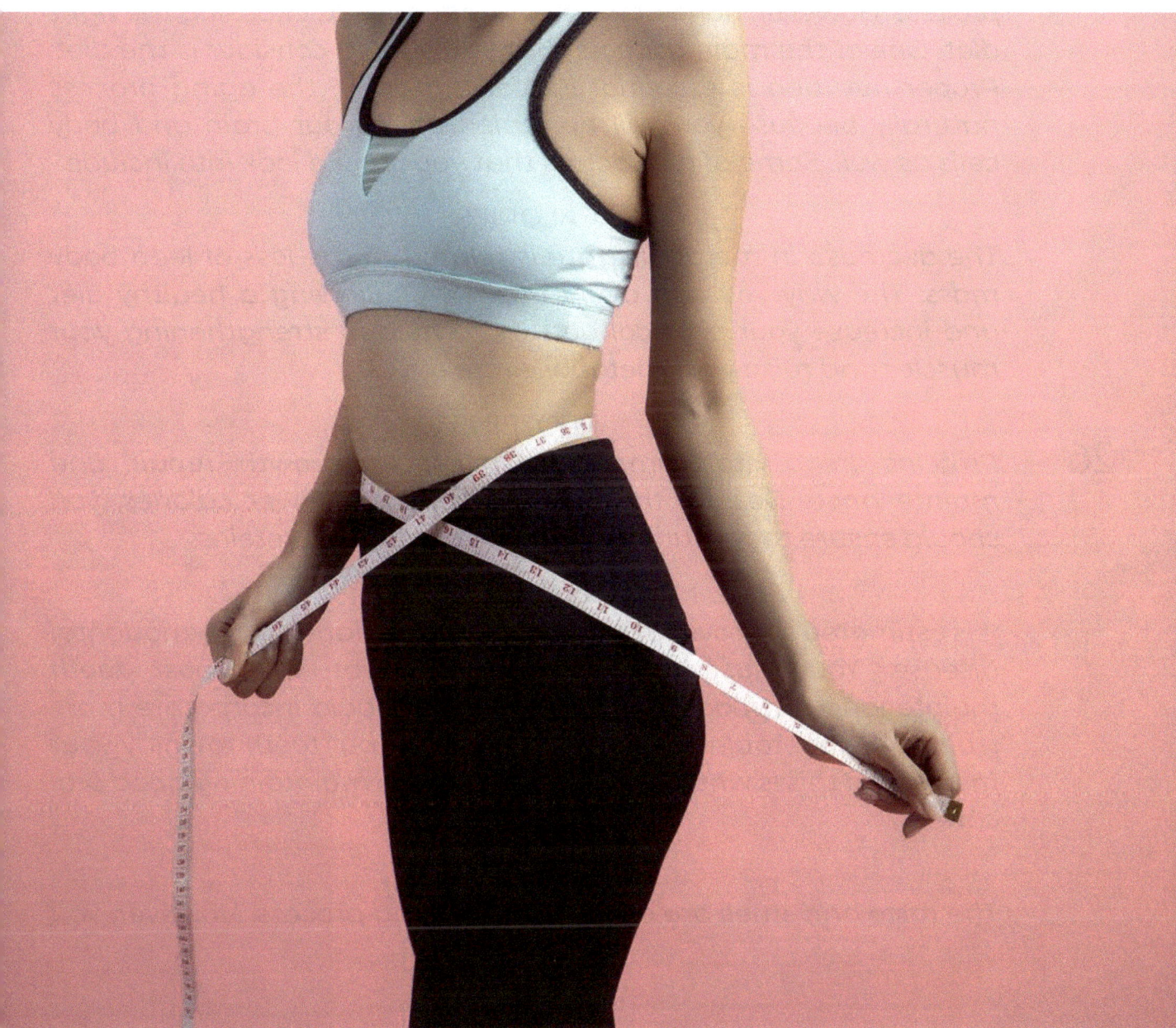

HOW PROPER NUTRITION HELPS SLOW DOWN AGING

Some products are promoted as ways to slow or prevent the aging process. However, none of them is as effective as choosing the right diet. One of the main aspects that you should consider is the diet. Proper nutrition is essential in slowing down the aging process naturally because you will be replenishing your brain and body cells as well. Some of the factors that you should look into include:

CALORIES

The decrease in metabolic rate is related to the loss of lean body mass. The way you can avoid this is by following a healthy diet and increase your physical activity to help in strengthening your muscles and raise your metabolic rate.

PROTEINS

26

Proteins are a vital component in cellular growth, repair, and maintenance. Despite the need to consume lower calories, you should ensure that your nutrition has adequate proteins.

DENTAL HEALTH

It is estimated that over 81% of the adult population has periodontal disease. You must observe nutrition that will boost teeth maintenance or foods with fluoride. You should incorporate more fruits and vegetables. You should have all your teeth to enjoy your meals, and this is where you should focus on maintaining good oral care.

TASTE

The taste and smell are dulled by the aging process. However, you can revamp it by staying hydrated throughout and resisting the use of a salt shaker. You can use herbs to enhance flavor in foods.

ANTIOXIDANTS

Antioxidants are essential nutritional components that slow down the aging process. The antioxidants can help in preventing chronic diseases.

CALCIUM AND VITAMIN D

The majority of the body requires calcium ions and vitamin D as we age. The mineral is essential for the proper functioning of the nervous system, blood clotting, and muscle contractions. Adequate calcium intake is essential in slowing down the aging process. In addition to the nutrients, you should always take an adequate amount of water to prevent dehydration and loss of vital chemicals.

27

28

Chapter 03

The Science Behind It

To bring the body into a ketogenic condition, you need to follow a high-fat diet and small carbohydrates without any grains, or almost any. The composition will be roughly 80% fat and 20% protein. For the very first two days, that will be the rule.

You need to eat a high-fat diet and minimal carbs without any grains, or almost any, to bring the body into a ketogenic condition. The composition would be about 80% fat and 20% protein. This will be the law for the very first two days.

When the body absorbs carbs, it induces an insulin surge that has the insulin emitted by the pancreas, and common sense assures us that if we then eliminate carbs, the insulin does not hold excess calories as the perfect fat. The body today has no carbs as an energy source, so your body should look for a new source.

29

If you decide to remove extra weight, this works well. The body must break down the extra fat and function with it, rather than carbs, as energy.

That particular condition is known as Ketosis. This is the state in which you want the body to be in, can make great sense when you want to drop excess fat while keeping muscle.

Yeah, now on to the portion of the diet and how to prepare it. With every pound of lean mass, you would need to ingest no less than one gram of protein. It will aid with strengthening and restoring muscle tissue during exercises & that kind of. Thinking ratio? 65% protein and 30% fat.

Effectively if you weigh 150 pounds, that means 150 g of protein a day. X4 (number of calories equivalent to 600 calories in a gram of protein); Any of the calories will come from fat. If the caloric maintenance is 3000, you need to consume about 500, less that might imply that one day if you require 2500 calories, about 1900 calories should come from the fats!

To fuel the body, you have to consume fats, which in exchange will also burn up excess fat! That is the diet plan rule; you've got to consume fats! The downside of taking healthy fats and the keto diet is you're not going to be thirsty. Fat processing of food is slow, operating to the benefit and making you feel whole.

30

You're going to be working on Monday-Friday, and then on the other days, you're going to have a "carb-up." The carb up starts on Friday with the last exercise, post-training, you need to take a liquid carbohydrate with your whey shake. This will help produce an insulin surge, which also allows us to provide the carbohydrates that the body urgently requires for restoring muscle mass and for glycogen stores to expand & refill.

Consume whatever you like during this specific process (carb up)- pizzas, crisps, spaghetti, ice cream. Somehow. This will be beneficial for you because it can refresh the body for the week ahead and provide the food that your body requires to nourish.

Switch your focus onto the no-carb high-fat average protein diet program as Sunday starts. Holding the body in Ketosis and losing fat is the optimal solution to get muscle.

An additional benefit of Ketosis is when you enter the ketosis state and burn the fat, the body will deplete from carbohydrates. Packing up with carbs can make you appear as full as before (but even with less body fat!), perfect for holiday activities if you visit the seaside or parties!

Let us recap on the diet schedule today:

•   Get in ketosis state by removing carbs and taking moderate/ low protein, high fat.

•   Take some kind of fiber to keep the pipes as clear as ever; you should realize what I mean.

•   If the ketosis protein consumption has been collected, per pound of lean mass will be no less than that of a g of protein.

So it is! It does require determination not to eat carbs during the week because certain products contain carbs; however, note that you would be greatly rewarded for the devotion.

You must not live on end days in Ketosis's condition because it is dangerous and will finish you; turning to make use of protein as a source of food is a no-no.

Ketogenic diet systems are structured primarily to trigger a ketosis condition within the body. If the volume of glucose within the body is low, the whole body turns to fat as a source of energy replacement.

The body has main sources of fuel, one of which is glucose. Free fatty acids (FFA) and, to a lesser degree, ketones from FFA Fat by-products are kept in the triglyceride type. Typically, they are split into long-chain fatty acids and glycerol.

The removal of glycerol from the triglyceride molecule enables the three free fatty acid (FFA) molecules to be used as energy for the introduction into the bloodstream.

The molecule of glycerol goes into the liver, where three molecules of it combine to create one molecule of sugar. Additionally, when the body consumes fat, it creates glucose as a by-product. Its glucose may be used to power different regions of the brain and body parts that can't operate on FFA molecules.

32

However, though glucose on its triglycerides will travel through the blood, cholesterol takes a carrier to go through the bloodstream. In a carrier known as LDL or low-density lipoprotein, cholesterol and triglycerides are packed. Thus, the larger the LDL particles, the greater the number of triglycerides it has.

The general process of energy-burning of fat deposits produces co2, oxygen, and ketone-known components. The liver produces ketones out of the free essential fatty acids. Right now, they consist of two classes of atoms joined by a purposeful carbonyl unit.

The body cannot shop ketones, and therefore they should be used or excreted at times. The body often excretes them as acetone through the breath and as acetoacetate through the urine.

The ketones may be used as a source of energy for body cells. The subconscious will use ketones to generate between 70-75 percent of the energy requirement.

As for alcoholic drinks, ketones take priority over carbohydrates as food resources. That means that they should be consumed first when filled with the bloodstream before glucose can be used as a fuel.

33

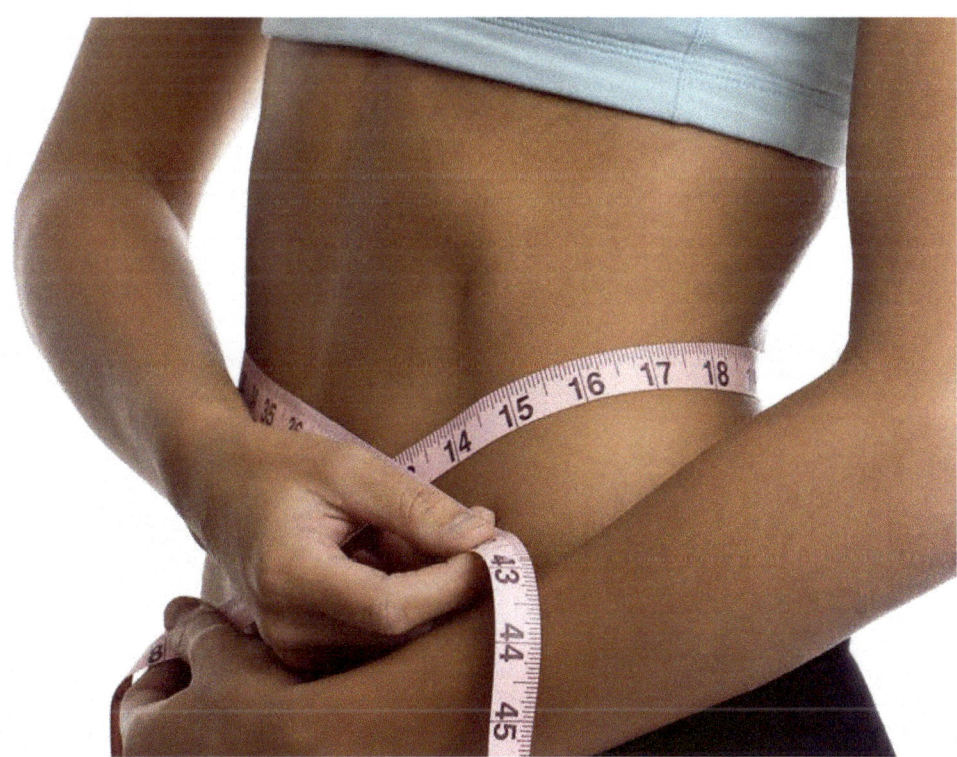

34

Chapter 04

Benefits of Ketogenic Diet for People Over 50

Unfortunately, one of the main aspects that you will not be able to eat whatever you want when you are following a keto diet. However, like many diets, you will have a wide array of options to choose from. You can find alternatives that you can enjoy and avoid a high carbohydrate diet. The essence of the keto diet is to get your body into ketosis, and all you need to do is to reduce your carbohydrate intake. Carbohydrates are not only the junk foods that you love but also some other healthier foods that you enjoy.

THE MACROS I SHOULD AIM FOR ON THE KETO DIET AFTER 50

Macro is a term that is coined from macronutrients, which include protein, fats, and carbohydrates, which makes up the composition of macronutrients required by the body. You can easily find this information listed on the nutritional facts panel of most foods, and you can use counting apps or calculators to calculate your macros. Gram for gram, the macronutrients are critical in the total calorie count that you will consume per day. One gram of carbohydrate will provide four calories; one gram of protein provides four calories, while one gram of fat will give you nine calories. Alcohol is also considered a macronutrient, and it gives seven calories per gram, although it has no nutritional value to the body.

When you follow your macro diet, you will go beyond counting calories, and you will focus more on macros. Depending on your

35

health objectives, you can adjust the ratios of the macronutrients that you consume to help you build muscle, lose weight, or enter a maintenance mode. If you follow a ketogenic diet, you will pay attention to net carbohydrates as part of the macros because it will determine how many useful carbohydrates you will consume per meal.

The macronutrients mustn't be confused with micronutrients, which are the key vitamins and minerals in the body. The micronutrients are required in small quantities, and they are essential in doing everything from regulating hormones to boosting brain performance. Macros are also different from the macrobiotic diet, which has principles drawn from Zen Buddhism.

KETO DIET MACROS BETWEEN MEN AND WOMEN AFTER 50

Macros zero in on the composition of your daily calories so that you can alter each to give you the best health that you want. If you have 70% calories in carbs, then you will feel different, unlike when you have 70% calories from fats. Men and women after 50 have to understand their macros so that they can adjust them according to their health and energy needs. With tracking, you can understand the source of the imbalance and make changes that will promote better growth and development of new cells.

Many people on a ketogenic diet will make the mistake of counting calories alone. This will not give them meaningful results because you will not know the balance of your energy source. If you want a more productive approach, you should monitor your macronutrients because it will tell you a more decent and better approach that you can use to achieve your health goals. Besides, when you follow the quality of your macros, you can potentially increase your fat-burning abilities and have a lean body.

HOW CALORIES RESTRICTION SLOWS DOWN AGING

For anyone who has never tracked their calories and learned the quality ratio of protein, fat, and carbohydrates that are effective for their body, it can be unusual. When you monitor your calories for a few days, you will know what your body needs and what you can do to enhance your health. You need a diet that will give you adequate energy throughout the day and boost cellular regeneration. There are reasons why the restriction of calories will slow down the aging process. Some of the benefits of calorie restriction include:

FLEXIBILITY AND CUSTOMIZATION

37

There is no one size fits all macros because everyone has their health objectives. However, when you choose the best calorie intake that will put your health goals forward, you will be able to make the right decision and reduce the cellular aging process. It is important to understand that cells age when they are not rejuvenated properly. When you restrict calories and choose one which improves cellular division, you will remain youthful.

HAVE MORE BALANCE IN YOUR DIET

Unlike other restrictive diets, you can monitor your calories and still enjoy the foods that you love. A ketogenic diet will reduce fat deposits in the peripheral and visceral organs, which often causes obesity, among other conditions. When your macronutrients are balanced, you will always feel energized and rejuvenated.

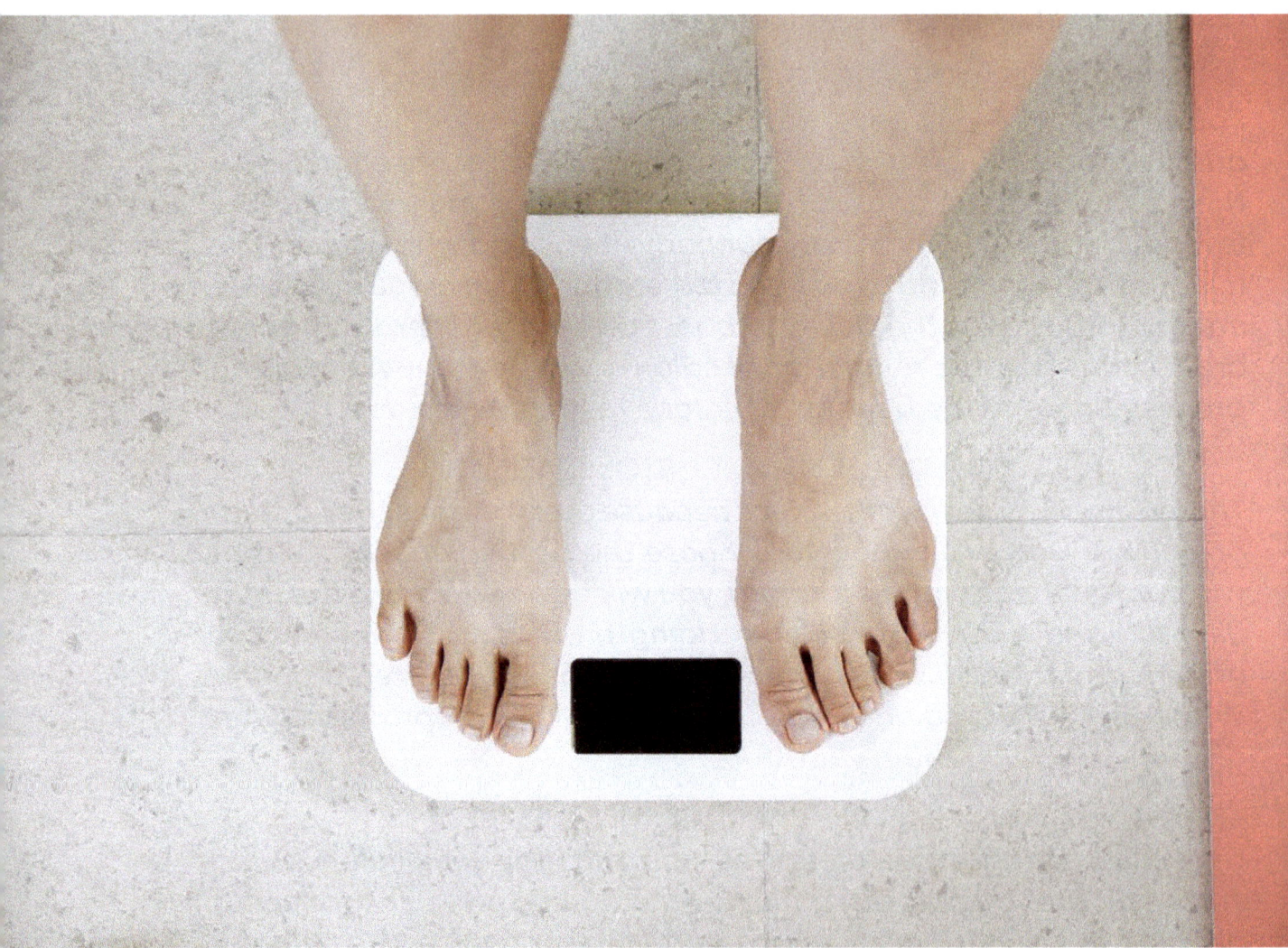

EASILY MANAGE MEDICAL CONDITIONS

Some studies indicate that managing your calorie intake is essential in building a better feeling and rejuvenation. Studies indicate that the macronutrients will help you manage conditions such as diabetes, polycystic ovary syndrome, and certain cancers. You must consult your physician before cutting down your calories.

HOW AGING AFFECTS YOUR NUTRITIONAL NEEDS

Nutrition is vital in maintaining a healthy biological system. You can lead a happy and fulfilling life when you choose the right nutrition. However, it is imperative to understand that nutrition changes with age, and if you are suffering from nutritional deficiencies, then it will bring harmful outcomes. In the initial years of childhood, the little bodies will require essential nutrients to enable them to grow and develop quickly, both physically and mentally. The food should provide high energy as well as nourishing capabilities that can enhance the cognitive abilities of the child. It is also important to note that the child is learning new foods and developing their taste, which will shape their eating habits in the future. Therefore, the kids should be encouraged to consume a wide array of foods to help them get all the essential nutrients. The key nutrient includes proteins necessary for growth, Vitamin D to help in the growth of strong bones. Along with other vital nutrients such as vitamin A are vital in boosting the immune system, while zinc and iron are essential in boosting the mental abilities of the kids.

During adolescence, 13-19 years, the body is going around significant

39

changes emotionally and physically because of puberty. Moreover, they are maturing now, and the growth of bones and muscles occurs during this phase. For this reason, you will require a diet that is rich in calcium, hence the importance of milk products. Iron is also an important component, and it can be obtained from meat, chicken, kidney beans, and spinach. During the teenage years, the body requires vital nutrients. Although many kids will want to switch to sugary foods and drinks, you should always encourage them to eat healthy foods because it will impact their life later.

Adulthood: 20 to 50 years, presents a myriad of challenges, and this is a time where you are required to maintain a healthy balance in the foods that you consume. The body cells are degenerating faster than they are being replaced hence the need to switch to a healthier diet and always consider your medical conditions. You should get enough nutrition of proteins, carbohydrates, and vitamins, as well as micronutrients. You must focus on a diet that will help you feel great without disturbing your body in terms of weight and emotional aspects. You need the energy to carry out your activities hence the need to balance your diet effectively.

40

Old age occurs when you are over 50 years, the body will need more vitamins, minerals, and proteins to help in building the cellular structure as well as maintain a good balance emotionally. The body's ability to absorb certain nutrients diminishes as you go past 50 years, and it is therefore important that you choose a diet that will replenish your nutrients regularly. If you are taking a diet that *does not have all the essential minerals and vitamins, then you should consider adding supplements to your diet. You should look at your body needs by monitoring the calories and macros because this will give you the best emotional and body balance.*

HOW PROPER NUTRITION HELPS SLOW DOWN AGING

Some products are promoted as ways to slow or prevent the aging process. However, none of them is as effective as choosing the right diet. One of the main aspects that you should consider is the diet. Proper nutrition is essential in slowing down the aging process naturally because you will be replenishing your brain and body cells as well. Some of the factors that you should look into include:

CALORIES

The decrease in metabolic rate is related to the loss of lean body mass. The way you can avoid this is by following a healthy diet and increase your physical activity to help in strengthening your muscles and raise your metabolic rate.

41

PROTEINS

Proteins are a vital component in cellular growth, repair, and maintenance. Despite the need to consume lower calories, you should ensure that your nutrition has adequate proteins.

DENTAL HEALTH

It is estimated that over 81% of the adult population has periodontal disease. You must observe nutrition that will boost teeth maintenance or foods with fluoride. You should incorporate more fruits and vegetables. You should have all your teeth to enjoy your meals, and this is where you should focus on maintaining good oral care.

TASTE

The taste and smell are dulled by the aging process. However, you can revamp it by staying hydrated throughout and resisting the use of a salt shaker. You can use herbs to enhance flavor in foods.

ANTIOXIDANTS

Antioxidants are essential nutritional components that slow down the aging process. The antioxidants can help in preventing chronic diseases.

CALCIUM AND VITAMIN D

The majority of the body requires calcium ions and vitamin D as we age. The mineral is essential for the proper functioning of the nervous system, blood clotting, and muscle contractions. Adequate calcium intake is essential in slowing down the aging process. In addition to the nutrients, you should always take an adequate amount of water to prevent dehydration and loss of vital chemicals.

42

Chapter 05

Ketogenic for Women Over 50 and How Ketogenic Benefits Them

The health benefits of the Keto diet are not different for men or women, but the speed at which they are reached does differ. As mentioned, women's bodies are a lot other when it comes to the ways that they can burn fats and lose weight. For example, by design, women have at least 10% more body fat than men. Don't be hard on yourself if you notice that it seems like men can lose weight easier—that's because they can! What women have in additional body fat, men typically have the same in muscle mass. This is why men tend to see faster external results because that added muscle mass means that their metabolism rates are higher. That increased metabolism means that fat and energy get burned faster. When you are on Keto, though, the internal change is happening right away.

43

As we age, we naturally look for ways to hold onto our youth and energy. It's not uncommon to think about things that promote anti-aging. Products and lifestyle changes are advertised everywhere, and they are designed to catch your attention as you grapple with the reality of what it means to be a 50+-year-old woman in our society. Even if you aren't eating for anti-aging yet, you have likely thought about it in terms of the way you treat your skin and hair, for example.

For instance, indigestion becomes as common as you age. This is because the body cannot break down certain foods like it used to. With all of the additives and fillers, we all become used to putting our bodies through discomfort in an attempt to digest regular meals. You are probably not even aware that you are doing this to your body, but upon trying a Keto diet, you will realize how your digestion will begin to change. You will no longer feel bloated or uncomfortable after you eat. If you notice this as a familiar feeling, you are likely not eating food that is nutritious enough to satisfy your needs and is only resulting in excess calories.

Keto fills you up in all of the ways that you need, allowing your body to digest and metabolize all of the nutrients truly. When you eat your meals, you should not feel the need to overeat to overcompensate for not having enough nutrients. Anything that takes stress off of any system in your body is going to become a form of anti-aging. You will quickly find this benefit once you start your Keto journey, as it is one of the first-reported changes that most participants notice. In addition to a healthier digestive system, you will also experience more regular bathroom usage, with little to none of the problems often associated with age.

While weight loss is one of the more common desires for most 50+ women who start a diet plan, the way that the weight is lost matters. If you have ever shed a lot of weight before, you have probably experienced the adverse effects of sagging or drooping skin that you were left to deal with. Keto rejuvenates the elasticity in your skin. Instead of having to do copious amounts of exercise to firm up your skin, it should already be becoming firmer each day that you are on the Keto diet. This is something that a lot of participants are

44

pleasantly surprised to find out.

Women also commonly report a natural reduction in wrinkles and healthier skin and hair growth, in general. Many women who start the diet report that they notice reverse effects in their aging process. While the skin becomes healthier and more supple, it also becomes firmer. Even if you aren't presently losing weight, you will still be able to appreciate the effects that Keto brings to your skin and face. Because your internal systems are becoming healthier by the day, this tends to show on the outside in a short amount of time. You will also begin to feel healthier. While it is possible to read about the experiences of others, there is nothing like feeling this for yourself when you start Keto.

Everyone, especially women over 50, has day-to-day tasks that are draining and require specific amounts of energy to complete. Aging can, unfortunately, take away from your energy reserve, even if you get enough sleep at night. It limits the way that you have to live your life, and this can become a very frustrating realization. Most diet plans bring about a sluggish feeling that you are simply supposed to get used to, for example. But Keto does the exact opposite. When you change your eating habits to fit the Keto guidelines, you are going to be hit with a boost of energy. Since your body is genuinely getting everything that it needs nutritionally, it will repay you with a sustained energy supply.

Another common complaint about women over 50 is that seemingly overnight, your blood sugar levels are going to be more sensitive

45

than usual. While everyone must keep an eye on these levels, it is especially necessary for those who are in their 50s and beyond. High blood sugar can be an indication that diabetes is on the way, but Keto can become a preventative measure that we've already talked about. Additionally, naturally regulating elevated blood sugar levels also reduces systemic inflammation, which is also common for women over 50. By balancing the immune system, of which inflammation is a part of, everyday aches and pains are reduced. Inflammation can also affect vital organs and is a precursor to cancer. Keto will support your path to an anti-inflammatory lifestyle.

There are a lot of benefits to starting a ketogenic diet for women after 50, be it in terms of weight, experience, or to improve your health!

46

LOSS AND MAINTENANCE OF WEIGHT

Gaining extra pounds (especially around the abdomen) and struggling with controlling the weight are common nuisances that menopausal and post-menopausal women have to deal with. As you can already imagine, this age-related problem is also a result of the decline in estrogen levels.

GOING KETO CAN HELP YOU LOSE WEIGHT AND BURN FAT IN A COUPLE OF WAYS

Going Keto Decreases Your Appetite –When your body gets used to filling up on fat and ditches the carbs, you will notice a severe decline in appetite. You will feel full for many hours after your meals, and you will keep your cravings at bay. The automatic decrease in appetite is one of the most significant benefits of the Keto diet.

GOING KETO LEADS TO RAPID WEIGHT LOSS

If you want to shed pounds in a matter of days, then going Keto is the best way to do it. Once you shift to fat for energy, a change in your body is about to happen. Once you have a decreased level of insulin, this hormone will give your kidneys an order to start eliminating the extra amounts of water from your body, which will leave you with a few pounds less, even after the first 7-10 days after choosing this diet.

CONTROL OF GLUCOSE IN THE BODY

Science has found out that decreased estrogen levels can promote insulin resistance, and in turn, increase blood sugar. When you have insulin resistance, your body is practically immune to the effects of insulin.

47

A REDUCTION IN RELIANCE ON THE MEDICATIONS-RELATED TO DIABETES

With Keto, you drastically limit your carbs and sugars consumption. With little blood sugar, your body does not need to release insulin to manage it. Thus, you prevent developing diabetes symptoms. If you already have it, the diet helps you to order it.

CONTROL OF HIGH BLOOD PRESSURE

Once you attain 50, you must monitor your blood pressure rates. Reduction in the intake of carbohydrates is a proven way to lower your blood pressure. When you cut down on your carbs and lower your blood sugar levels, you significantly reduce your chances of getting other diseases.

AN IMPROVED MENTAL PERFORMANCE

The Keto diet provides your body and brain with a stable fuel source—ketones. The diet prevents sugar swings that are associated with a carb-rich diet. That allows you to avoid brain fog, improves your focus, concentration, and mental clarity.

RESTORATION OF INSULIN SENSITIVITY

That is the first objective of a Keto diet. It helps stabilize the insulin levels and thereby improve fat burning. Using a Keto diet helps preserve your muscles while burning fat in your body.

48

IMPROVE CHOLESTEROL LEVELS

It will help reduce blood cholesterol levels by consuming fewer carbohydrates while on the Keto diet. That is due to the increased lipolysis condition. That leads to lower levels of LDL cholesterol and higher levels of HDL cholesterol.

SATIETY

Eating protein reduces the ghrelin (the hunger hormone) and stimulates the production of the satiety hormones. When you eat protein, it's transformed into amino acids, which help your body with various processes such as building muscle and regulating immune function.

EFFECTIVE IN FIGHTING EPILEPSY

The primary goal of this diet, introduced in Antiquity, was to fight against epilepsy. The ketones may affect anti-convulsion, but to date, it is not possible to say why they have this effect on the body.

Without going too far into the scientific part, ketone bodies would have an impact on the concentrations of glutamate and GABA (Gamma-Amino Butyric Acid). Glutamate is the main excitatory neuro-mediator of the central nervous system, and GABA, the main inhibitory neuro-mediator. This would explain why the ketogenic diet has such essential effects on people with epilepsy. But I don't want to lose you with my scientific explanations; you can do your research if the subject interests you.

EFFECTIVE IN TYPE I OR TYPE II DIABETES

49

Diabetes results from a problem in the metabolism of carbohydrates. Therefore, the diet is naturally a place to relieve the signs and symptoms in a person with diabetes, whether for type I or type II diabetes. Whether the problem is a defect in insulin production or insulin resistance, the ketogenic diet will make it possible to get around the problem.

When you are Keto-adapted, your blood sugar drops sharply because you only eat foods low in carbohydrates. The ketogenic diet can, therefore, allow you to control your blood sugar, which can be very useful in managing your diabetes. The ketogenic diet will allow you to reduce your insulin levels to healthy and stable values.

EFFECTIVE IN PEOPLE WITH ALZHEIMER'S

Excuse me in advance, but in this part, we will tackle a scientific "hair" side to explain the benefits of the ketogenic diet in the treatment of Alzheimer's disease.

In addition to all this, the ketogenic diet would have a role in protecting against oxidative stress, and therefore would be preventive and effective against cell death. This would, therefore, limit brain degeneration.

IMPROVES CONCENTRATION

The ketones are an excellent source of fuel for the brain. As you decrease your carbohydrate intake, you avoid blood sugar spikes, which often appear after meals. This allows your body to prevent focusing on eliminating carbohydrates and concentrate on the activity you are doing.

50

OTHER BENEFITS OF KETOGENIC DIETS

- *Appetite control*

- *Lowers your risk of heart disease*

- *More energy and improved mental performance*

- *Boosts brain functions*

- *Helps to reduce the risk of cancer*

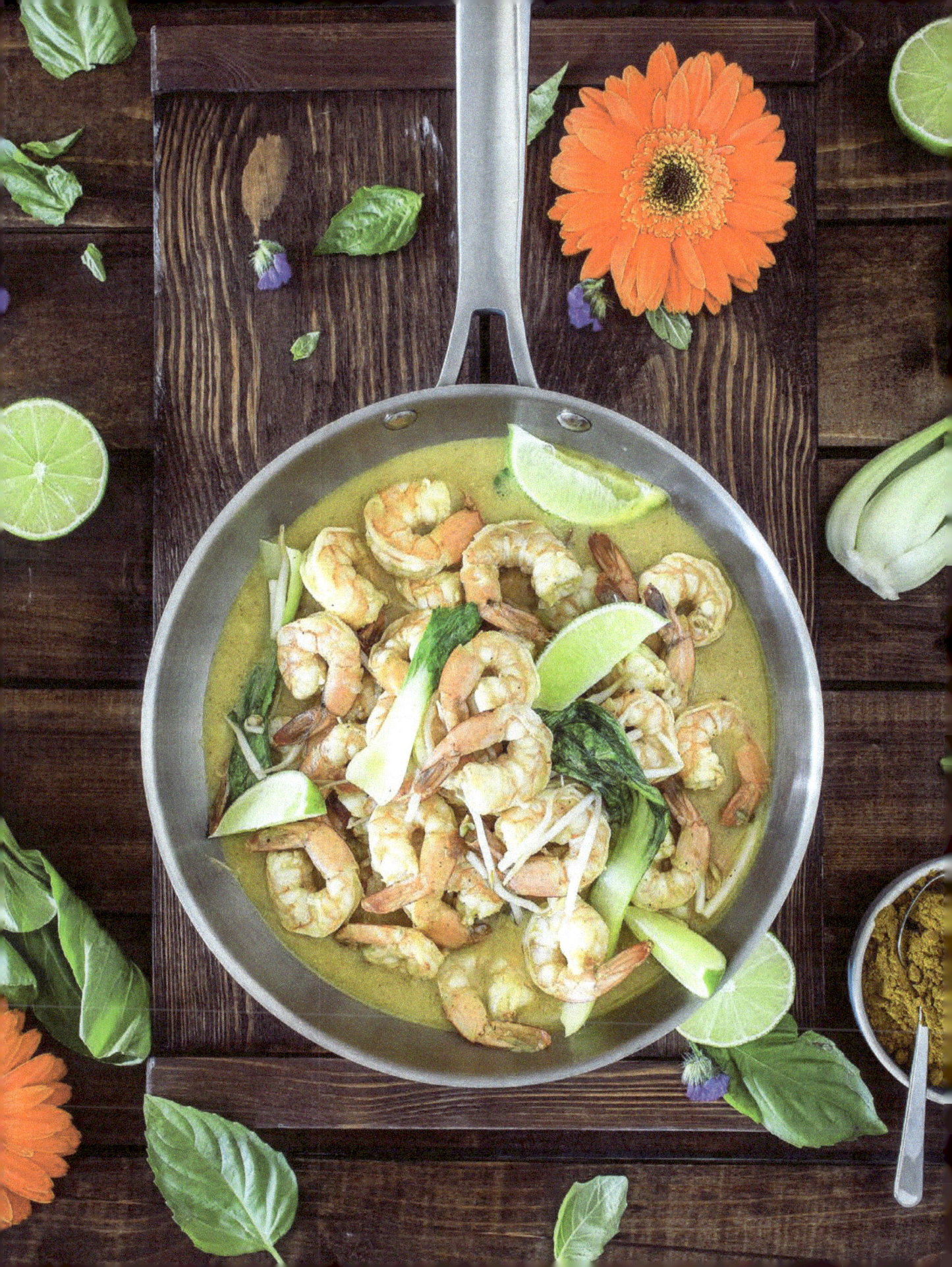

52

Chapter 06

How to Start a Keto Diet After 50 and Understanding How to Calculate Net Carbs

A FEW PROPOSALS THAT MAY ASSIST YOU WITH YOUR OBJECTIVES ON A KETO DIET

To start with, ensure that you're following something beyond your carbs. Keto is minimal in carb (20g or less every day as you're as of now doing), yet it has moderate protein (50–75 grams for every day for ladies) and high fat (in any event a 1:1 up to a 1:2 proportion of protein to fat). In case you're not previously following your protein and fat alongside your carbs, start.

The protein and fat are particularly significant in case you're attempting to get "ripped," as you state. You need the protein to construct muscle and the fat to give you vitality to work out.

Keep in mind, on Keto you're changing your body from consuming carbs and sugars for fuel to using body fats for energy—which is better for your body, your brain, and for work out. However, in case you're not giving enough fats for your body, you won't have sufficient energy to consume.

Furthermore, since you express that you've generally been thin, you likely don't have a lot, assuming any, you need an abundance of fat on your body to consume, so you certainly need to get the fat in your nourishment consistently.

Second, you state that you're on a considerable shortfall. You most likely don't have to follow your calories at all in case you're eating

53

Keto effectively. Keto depends on tuning in to your body—eating when you're eager and halting eating when you're full.

This sounds basic; however, it conflicts with what most of us have learned and done for our entire lives—eating three suppers every day at recommended times and cleaning our plates whether we're ravenous. What's more, since you'll be eating significantly more fat than the amount used to and not a lot of carbs by any stretch of the imagination (which causes desires and sugar crashes), you'll feel full quicker. For more, so you won't eat to such an extent, and you won't have any desire to eat as frequently, which implies the calories will deal with themselves. (Numerous individuals on the keto diet just eat a couple of suppers daily since they simply aren't ravenous more than that.)

54

For you explicitly, since you're attempting to pick up muscle and you're as of now thin, you unquestionably don't should be on a calorie-confined or calorie shortage diet—and you may need to eat close to the top finish of the protein to fat proportion to ensure your body has the vitality it needs. So, eat that great fat and protein and appreciate them!

Third, one of the general most significant advantages of Keto is getting your body into ketosis—which is the consequence of changing your body from consuming carbs and sugars to consuming fats. For competitors, this is fundamental with the goal that you can have the most elevated conceivable execution. When your body is in ketosis, you'll notice numerous advantages that will assist you with your exhibition—more vitality, better rest, more stamina, and so forth. So, it's incredibly significant that you see all the segments of the keto method for eating with the goal that you can get your body into ketosis.

For more insights regarding eating Keto, look at this asset, CRACK the Keto CODE, which contains bunches of extraordinary information including the ideal nourishments on Keto. The food sources perfect for maintaining a strategic distance from, how to track (and change) your macros, what are electrolytes and for what reason are they so significant (particularly as a competitor this will be a serious deal for you), and even some incredible keto plans.

FASTING OR NOT FASTING

The topic of fasting is controversial. Indeed, fasting is good if it is done the correct way. Unreasonable fasting isn't acceptable.

55

An average individual ordinarily eats three suppers every day and snacks in the middle. The gastric discharging time after a healthy feast is 4 hours. Yet, before the nourishment is exhausted out, we nibble/eat more. We are continually keeping our digestive organs grinding away. Fasting allows our digestion tracts to rest. Also, there are many poisons created in our body, and they never find an opportunity to be purged.

Thirdly, it fortifies your body and improves resistance, for, during this period, you have washed down yourself, yet have ingested just simple squeezes that get retained no problem at all. You retain everything. Also, afterward, you feel spotless, sound, crisp, and revived. It sure is a great idea to watch a quick to detoxify yourself on more than one occasion per year.

Before we talk about something that gets the job done, could we stop for a minute and consider these crazy weight control plans we hear about? It appears each week the web has some new prevailing fashion diet, detox, or quick. If even 10% of the guarantees they make are genuine, we'd never need another again. Everybody swears their eating routine is the one which works. Everyone has their little snare.

People fast to get in shape. Others do fast to detox their bodies or for strict reasons. In case you're fasting to get in shape, you might need to reevaluate. The weight reduction may not last after you complete the process of fasting. On the off chance that you will likely detox your body, you should realize that your body detoxes itself typically.

WHY CAN FASTING FOR WEIGHT LOSS BACKFIRE

At the point when you eat short of what you need, and you get more fit, your body goes into starvation mode. Your digestion eases back down to spare vitality. At the point when you finish fasting and return to your standard eating regimen, you may recover the weight you lost, to say the very least.

On a fast, your body alters by checking your craving so that you will feel less eager from the start. Be that as it may, when you have quit fasting, you're craving fires up back. You may feel hungrier and be bound to indulge.

Fasting each day has comparative outcomes. It assists individuals with shedding pounds, yet not for long. Be that as it may, the weight reduction didn't last after some time.

FASTING SAFELY

Fasting for a couple of days likely won't hurt a great many people who are reliable if they don't get dried out. Yet, fasting for extended periods is awful for you.

Your body needs nutrients, minerals, and different supplements from nourishment to remain healthy. On the off chance that you don't get enough, you can have manifestations, for example, weakness, wooziness, blockage, drying out, and not having the option to endure cold temperatures. Fasting too long can be perilous. Try not to fast, in any event, for a brief timeframe, on the off chance that you have diabetes since it can prompt risky dunks and spikes in glucose. Others who shouldn't fast are ladies who are pregnant or breastfeeding, anybody with a chronic disease, the old, and kids.

57

Before you go on another eating regimen, especially one that includes fasting, inquire as to whether it's a decent decision for you. You can likewise approach your primary care physician for a referral to an enrolled dietitian, who can tell you the best way to structure a smart dieting plan.

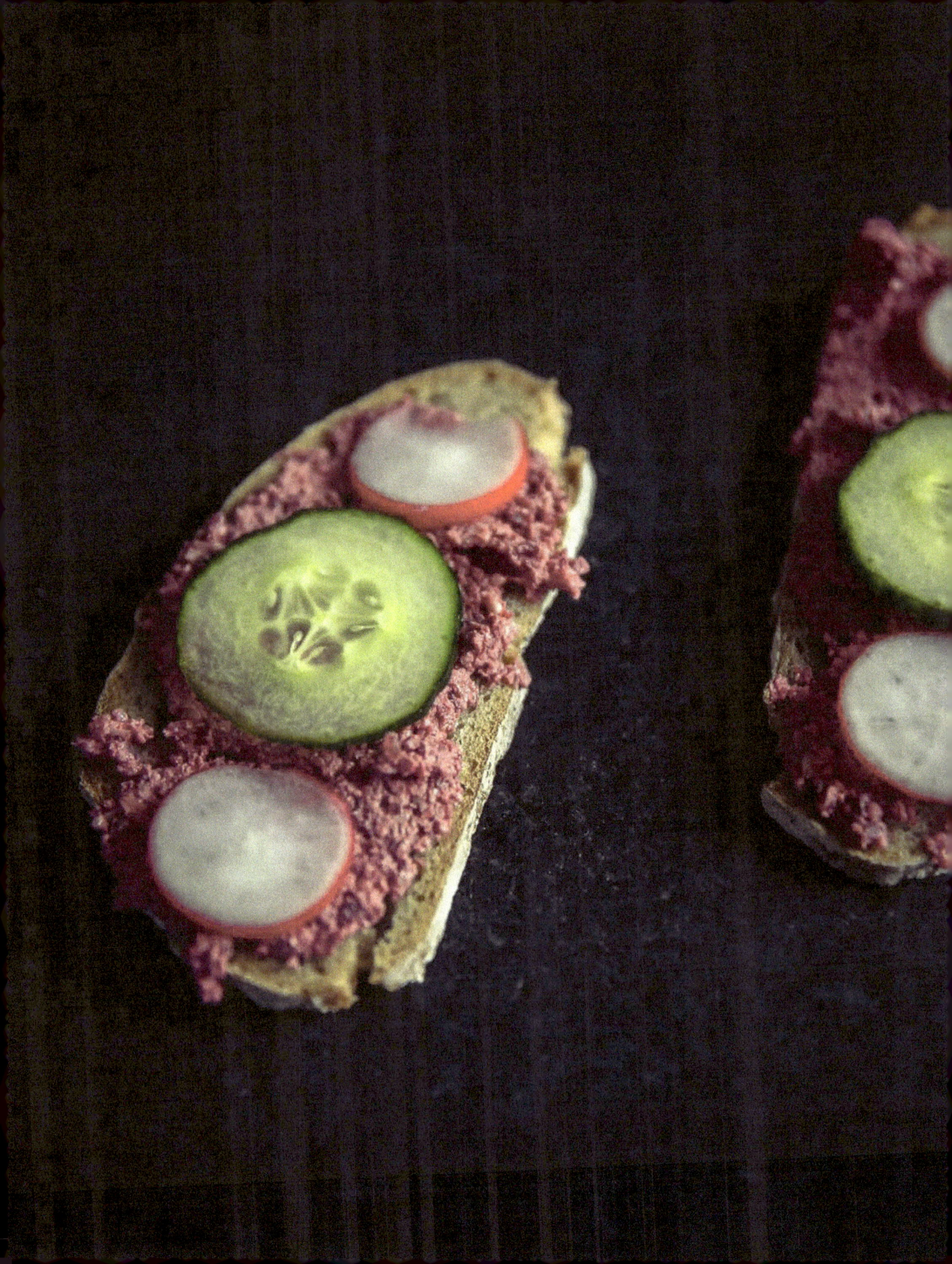

Chapter 07

Common Mistakes Seniors Make While Starting Keto

Do you feel like you are giving your all to the keto diet, but you still aren't seeing the results you want? You are measuring ketones, working out, and counting your macros, but you still aren't losing the weight you want. Here are the most common mistakes that most people make when beginning the keto diet.

1. TOO MANY SNACKS

There are many snacks you can enjoy while following the keto diet, like nuts, avocado, seeds, and cheese. But snacking can be an easy way to get too many calories into the diet while giving your body an easy fuel source besides stored fat. Snacks need to be only used if you frequently hunger between meals. If you aren't extremely hungry, let your body turn to your stored fat for its fuel between meals instead of dietary fat.

59

2. NOT CONSUMING ENOUGH FAT

The ketogenic diet isn't all about low carbs. It's also about high fats. You need to be getting about 75 percent of your calories from healthy fats, five percent from carbs, and 20 percent from protein. Fat makes you feel fuller longer, so if you eat the correct amount, you will minimize your carb cravings, and this will help you stay in ketosis. This will help your body burn fat faster.

3. CONSUMING EXCESSIVE CALORIES

You may hear people say you can eat what you want on the keto diet as long as it is high in fat. Even though we want that to be true, it is very misleading. Healthy fats need to make up the biggest part of your diet. If you eat more calories than what you are burning, you will gain weight, no matter what you eat, because these excess calories get stored as fat. An average adult only needs about 2,000 calories each day, but this will vary based on many factors like activity level, height, and gender.

4. CONSUMING A LOT OF DAIRIES

For many people, dairy can cause inflammation and keeps them from losing weight. Dairy is a combo food meaning it has carbs, protein, and fats. If you eat a lot of cheese as a snack for the fat content, you are also getting a dose of carbs and protein with that fat. Many people can tolerate dairy, but moderation is the key. Stick with no more than one to two ounces of cheese or cream at each meal. Remember to factor in the protein content.

60

5. CONSUMING A LOT OF PROTEIN

The biggest mistake that most people make when just beginning the keto diet is consuming too much protein. Excess protein gets converted into glucose in the body called gluconeogenesis. This is a natural process where the body converts the energy from fats and proteins into glucose when glucose isn't available. When following a ketogenic diet, gluconeogenesis happens at different rates to keep body function. Our bodies don't need a lot of carbs, but we do need glucose. You can eat absolute zero carbs, and through gluconeogenesis, your body will convert other substances into glucose to be used as fuel. This is why carbs only make up five percent of your macros. Some parts of our bodies need carbs to survive, like the kidney, medulla, and red blood cells. With gluconeogenesis, our bodies make and stores extra glucose as glycogen just in case supplies become too low.

In a normal diet, when carbs are always available, gluconeogenesis happens slowly because the need for glucose is extremely low. Our body runs on glucose and will store excess protein and carbs as fat.

It does take time for our bodies to switch from using glucose to burning fats. Once you are in ketosis, your body will use fat as the main fuel source and will start to store excess protein as glycogen.

6. NOT GETTING ENOUGH WATER

Water is crucial for your body. Water is needed for all your body does, and this includes burning fat. If you don't drink enough water, it can cause your metabolism to slow down, and this can halt your weight loss. Drinking 64 ounces or one-half gallon every day will help your body burn fat, flush out toxins, and circulate nutrients. When you are just beginning the keto diet, you might need to drink more water since your body will begin to get rid of body fat by flushing it out through urine.

61

7. CONSUMING TOO MANY SWEETS

Some people might indulge in keto brownies and keto cookies that are full of sugar substitute just because their net carb content is low, but you have to remember that you are still eating calories. Eating sweets might increase your carb cravings. Keto sweets are great on occasion; they don't need to be a staple in the diet.

8. NOT GETTING ENOUGH SLEEP

Getting plenty of sleep is needed in order to lose weight effectively. Without the right amount of sleep, your body will feel stressed, and this could result in your metabolism slowing down. It might cause it to store fat instead of burning fat. When you feel tired, you are more tempted to drink more lattes for energy, eat a snack to give you an extra boost, or order takeout rather than cooking a healthy meal. Try to get between seven and nine hours of sleep each night. Understand that your body uses that time to burn fat without you even lifting a finger.

9. LOW ON ELECTROLYTES

62

Most people will experience the keto flu when you begin this diet. This happens for two reasons when your body changes from burning carbs to burning fat, your brain might not have enough energy, and this, in turn, can cause grogginess, headaches, and nausea. You could be dehydrated, and your electrolytes might be low since the keto diet causes you to urinate often.

Getting the keto flu is a great sign that you are heading in the right direction. You can lessen these symptoms by drinking more water or taking supplements that will balance your electrolytes.

10. CONSUMING HIDDEN CARBS

Many foods look like they are low carb, but they aren't. You can find carbs in salad dressings, sauces, and condiments. Be sure to check nutrition labels before you try new foods to make sure it doesn't have any hidden sugar or carbs. It just takes a few seconds to skim the label, and it might be the difference between whether or not you'll lose weight.

If you have successfully ruled out all of the above, but you still aren't losing weight, you might need to talk with your doctor to make sure you don't have any health problems that could be preventing your weight loss. This can be frustrating, but stick with it, stay positive, and stay in the game. When the keto diet is done correctly, it is one of the best ways to lose weight.

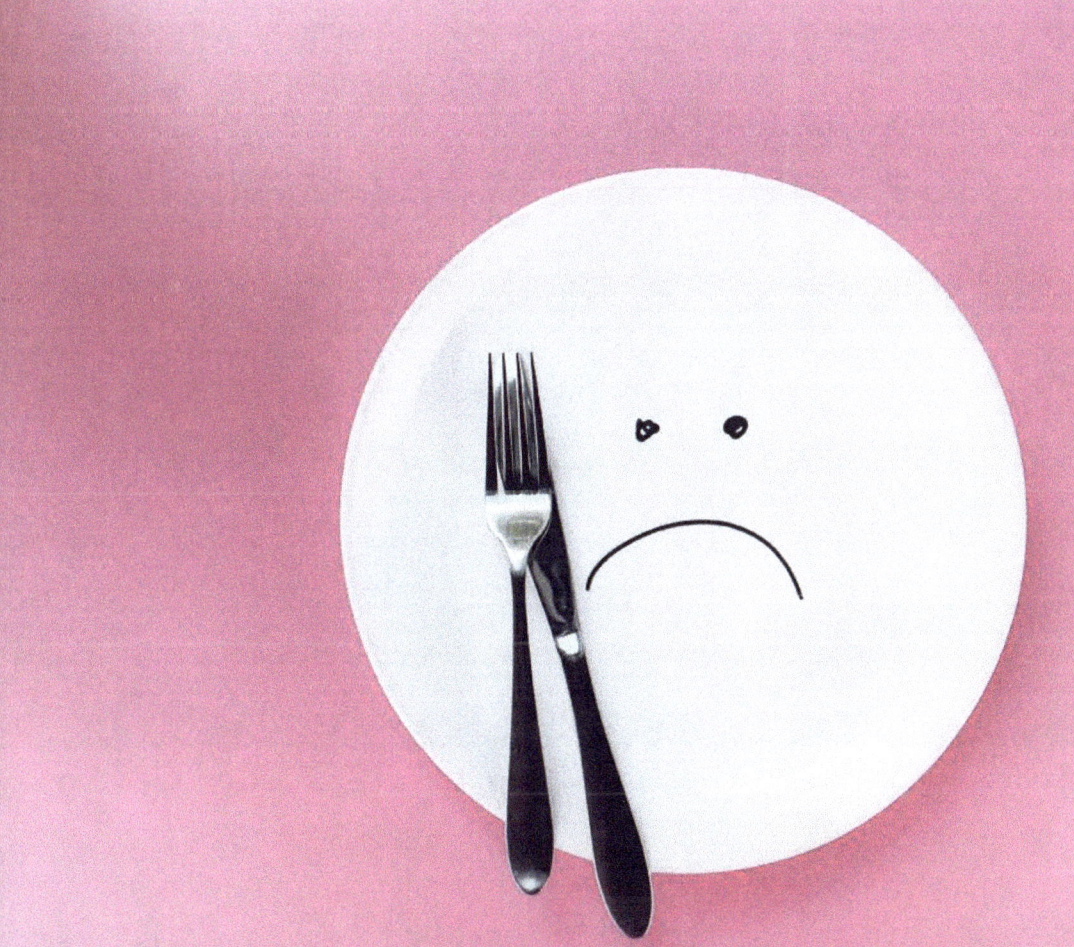

64

Chapter 08

Keto Tips for Seniors Who Want to Start

Routines are very important on this diet, and it's something that will help you stay healthy. As such, in this chapter, we are going to be giving you tips and tricks to make this diet work better for you and help you get an idea of routines that you can put in place for yourself.

Tip number one that is so important is DRINK WATER! This is absolutely vital for any diet that you're on, and you need it if not on one as well. However, this vital tip is crucial on a keto diet because when you are eating fewer carbs, you are storing less water, meaning that you are going to get dehydrated very easily. You should aim for more than the daily amount of water; however, remember that drinking too much water can be fatal as your kidneys can only handle so much as once. While this has mostly happened to soldiers in the military, it does happen to dieters as well, so it is something to be aware of.

65

Along with that same tip is to keep your electrolytes. You have three major electrolytes in your body. When you are on a keto diet, your body is reducing the amount of water that you store. It can be flushing out the electrolytes that your body needs as well, and this can make you sick. Some of the ways that you can fight this is by either salting your food or drinking bone broth. You can also eat pickled vegetables.

Eat when you're hungry instead of snacking or eating constantly.

This is also going to help, and when you focus on natural foods and healthy foods, this will help you even more. Eating processed foods is the worst thing you can do for fighting cravings, so you should really get into the routine of trying to eat whole foods instead.

Another routine that you can get into is setting a note somewhere that you can see it that will remind you of why you're doing this in the first place and why it's important to you. Dieting is hard, and you will have moments of weakness where you're wondering why you are doing this. Having a reminder will help you feel better, and it can really help with your perspective.

66

Tracking progress is something that straddles the fence. A Lot of people say that this helps a lot of people and you can celebrate your wins; however, as everyone is different and they have different goals, progress can be slower in some than others. This can cause others to be frustrated and sad, as well as wanting to give up. One of the most important things to remember is that while progress takes time, and you shouldn't get discouraged if you don't see results right away. With most diets, it takes at least a month to see any results. So, don't get discouraged and keep trying if your body is saying that you can. If you can't, then you will need to talk to your doctor and see if something else is for you.

You should make it a daily routine to try and lower your stress. Stress will not allow you to get into ketosis, which is that state that Keto wants to put you in. The reason for this being that stress increases the hormone known as cortisol in your blood, and it will prevent your body from being able to burn fats for energy. This is because your body has too much sugar in your blood. If you're going through a really high period of stress right now in your life, then this diet is not a great idea. Some great ideas for this would be getting into the habit or routine of taking the time to do something relaxing, such as walking and making sure that you're getting enough sleep, leads to the following routine that you need to do.

You need to get enough sleep. This is so important not just for your diet but also for your mind and body as well. Poor sleep also raises those stress hormones that can cause issues for you, so you need to get into the routine of getting seven hours of sleep at night on the minimum and nine hours if you can. If you're getting less than this, you need to change the routine you have in place right now and make sure that you establish a new routine where you are getting more sleep. As a result, your health and diet will be better.

67

Another routine that you need to get into is to give up diet soda and sugar substitutes. This is going to help you with your diet as well because diet soda can actually increase your sugar levels to a bad amount, and most diet sodas contain aspartame. This can be a carcinogen, so it's actually quite dangerous. Another downside is that using these sugar substitutes just makes you want more sugar. Instead, you need to get into the habit of drinking water or sparkling water if you like the carbonation.

Staying consistent is another routine that you need to get yourself into. No matter what you are choosing to do, make sure it's something that you can actually do. Try a routine for a couple of weeks and make serious notes of mental and physical problems that you're going through as well as any emotional issues that come your way. Make changes as necessary until you find something that works well for you and that you can stick to it. Remember that you need to give yourself time to get used to this and time to get used to changes before you give up on them.

Be honest with yourself, as well. This is another big tip for this diet. If you're not honest with yourself, this isn't going to work. Another reason that you need to be honest with yourself is if something isn't working, you need to be able to understand that and change it. Are you giving yourself enough time to make changes? Are you pushing too hard? If so, you need to understand what is going on with yourself and how you need to deal with the changes that you're going through. Remember not to get upset or frustrated. This diet takes time, and you need to be able to be a little more patient to make this work effectively.

68

Getting into the routine of cooking for yourself is also going to help you so much on this diet. Eating out is fun, but honestly, on this diet, it can be hard to eat out. It is possible to do so with a little bit of special ordering and creativity, but you can avoid all the trouble by simply cooking for yourself. It saves time, and it saves a lot of cash.

This subsequent topic falls into both the tip and routine category. Get into the habit of cleaning your kitchen. It's very hard to stick to a diet if your kitchen is dirty and full of junk food. Clear out the junk (donate it if you can, even though it's junk, there are tons of hungry people that would appreciate it) and replace all of the bad food with healthy keto food instead. Many people grab the carbs like crazy because they haven't cleared out their cabinets, and it's everywhere they look. Remember, with this diet, no soda, pasta, bread, candy, and things of that nature. Replacing your food with healthy food and making a regular routine of cleaning your kitchen and keeping the bad food out is going to help you be more successful with your diet, which is what you want here.

Getting into the routine of having snacks on hand is a good idea as well. This keeps you from giving in to temptation while you're out, and you can avoid reaching for that junk food. You can make sure that they are healthy, and you will be sticking to your high-intensity diet, which is what you want.

69

Try not to overeat as this will throw you out of where you need to be. Get into the routine of paying attention to what you're eating and how much. If this is something that you're struggling with, try investing in a food scale. You will be able to see what it is your eating precisely and make sure that you are understanding your portions, and making sure you stay in ketosis.

Another tip is to make sure that you're improving your gut health. This is so important. Your gut is pretty much linked to every other system in your body, so make sure that this something that you want to take seriously. When you have healthy gut flora, your body's hormones, along with your insulin sensitivity and metabolic *flexibility, will all be more efficient. When your flexibility is functioning at an optimal level, your body is able to adapt to your diet easier. If it's not, then it will convert the fat you are trying to use for energy into body fat.*

Batch cooking or meal prepping is another routine that is a good thing to get into. This is an especially good routine for on the go women. When you cook in batches, you are able to make sure that you have meals that are ready to go, and you don't have to cook every single day, and you can save a lot of time as well. You will also be making your environment better for your diet because you're supporting your goals instead of working against them.

The last tip is to mention exercise again. Getting into the routine of exercising can boost your ketone levels, and it can help you with your issues on transitioning to keto. The exercises also use different types of energy for the fuel you need. When your body gets rid of the glycogen storages, it needs other forms of energy, and it will turn into that energy that you need. Just remember to avoid exercises that are going to hurt you. Stay in the smaller exercises and lower intensity.

Following these tips and getting into these routines is going to help you stay on track and make sure that your diet will go as smoothly as it possibly can.

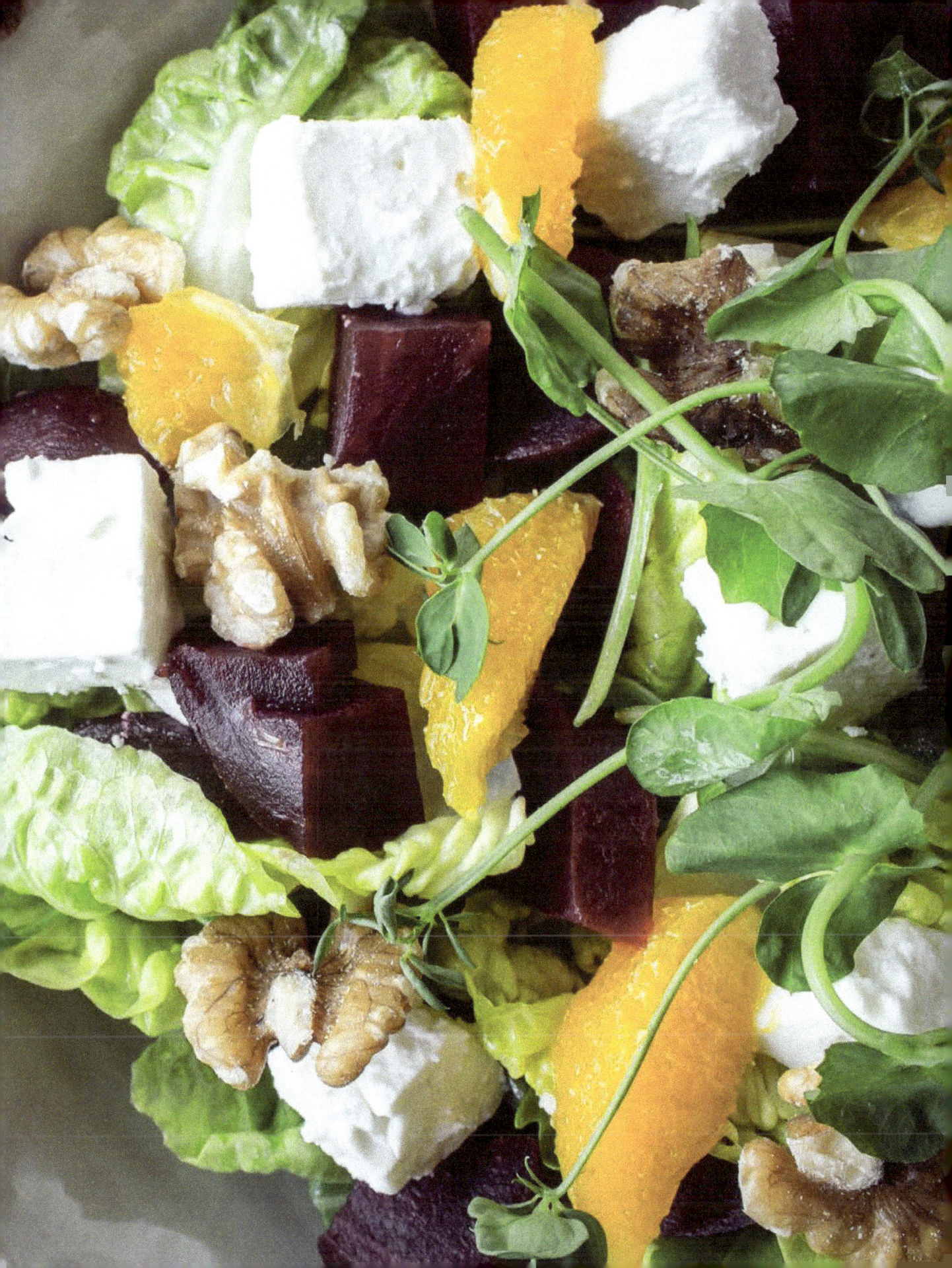

72

Chapter 09

Side Effects of Keto Diet and How to Solve Them

KETO BREATH

One of the most common side effects of a keto diet is bad breath. Not everyone who adopts the keto diet experiences this problem, but it is common. Bad breath comes as a result of internal metabolism processes. Your liver metabolizes the massive amounts of fat you are consuming and then converts them to ketone bodies such as acetone. These ketone bodies are broken down into smaller structures and are then circulated inside your body. As the ketone bodies circulate, they get into your lungs through the diffusion process, and eventually, exerted out through your breath.

HOW TO OVERCOME KETO BREATH

You can control bad keto breath by increasing water intake. You can also get rid of this problem by practicing good oral hygiene like regularly brushing your teeth. Alternatively, you can mask ketosis odor using mints and gums. It is also advisable to eat slightly more carbs and less protein if you have this problem.

73

KETO FLU

You may experience symptoms resembling those of flu, especially during your first days on a keto diet. Such symptoms include aches, fatigue, cramping, skin rash, and diarrhea. The side effects are caused by dehydration as a result of your body losing a lot of water and electrolytes.

When your body uses fat to fuel its functions instead of using protein, you tend to lose more water and electrolytes through urination. The loss of water and electrolytes is accelerated further by the low insulin levels and muscle glycogen that accompanies the keto diet.

Besides, most keto diets consist of food with little water and potassium levels, further accelerating the loss of body water and electrolytes.

HOW TO OVERCOME KETO FLU

You can handle keto flu by drinking a lot of water. You can also eat lots of soup. If you get enough rest, you will give your body enough energy to fight the flu on its own.

You need to lower the effects of keto flu by getting enough sleep. You can also drink a lot of water to minimize the impact of keto flu. There are also some supplements found in natural sources like organic coffee or matcha tea that could help you overcome the flu. Make a point to get enough salts and electrolytes, too.

74

FATIGUE

You may experience extreme feelings of tiredness once you adopt a keto diet. Fatigue is caused by a lack of glucose reaching your brain. Although this side effect will last for a few days, it could still cause much discomfort and worry on your part.

HOW TO OVERCOME KETO FATIGUE

Drink a lot of water and get enough rest. You can also avoid engaging in strenuous exercises. You can also eat healthy carbs to give you the extra energy your body needs.

GI SIDE EFFECTS

Keto diet can also harm your digestive system over the long term. Keto diet has been thought to cause some stomach problems such as constipation, high cholesterol levels, diarrhea, kidneys stones, and vomiting.

You may also experience abnormal stomach gas due to the sugar alcohols found in some keto diets, for example, the sugars found in some processed foods. The higher the amount of food you eat, the higher the impact of the side effects on you.

HOW TO CONTROL GI PROBLEMS WHEN YOU ARE ON A KETO DIET

Drink lots of water and eat high fiber foods such as fruits and vegetables to encourage the growth of beneficial bacteria in your GI system. Make it a habit of exercising regularly.

75

WEAKENED IMMUNE SYSTEM

Keto diets can also weaken the immune systems of some people. Studies suggest that keto foods could cause a condition called dysbiosis. Dysbiosis occurs when the balance of helpful and harmful bacteria is altered in your GI tract. The disruption is caused by the consumption of highly saturated fats and low fiber levels in your digestive system.

When you ingest diets with little prebiotic fiber, the number of beneficial bacteria decreases substantially in your digestive system. Your GI tract is the backbone of your immune system, and any compromise to it could have a negative impact on the immune functions leading to exposure to chronic diseases.

How to avoid weakened immune system when on a keto diet

Incorporate workouts into your keto diet. You can also eat high fiber food, such as fruits and vegetables. Also, ensure you drink lots of water.

VITAMIN AND OTHER MINERAL DEFICIENCIES

If you are on the keto diet, you may not receive enough vitamins and minerals needed for your body to function normally. Plant-based minerals such as calcium and vitamin D may not be present in your keto diet in the quantities required by your body. If these minerals decrease in your body for long periods, you may stand a high risk of getting lifestyle diseases such as heart failure.

Heart failure comes as a result of the hardening of your heart muscles because of the lack of enough selenium. Selenium is an essential immune-boosting antioxidant usually occurring in plant-based food. Lack of this critical antioxidant causes the hardening of your heart muscles leading to heart failure.

How to Treat the Deficiencies When You Are on a Keto Diet

Eat lots of fruits and vegetables to get vitamins. You can also use beneficial supplements to treat any deficiencies, which comes with the keto diet.

INCREASED RISK OF CHRONIC DISEASE

76

The Keto diet requires you to put a limit on the number of carbohydrates and protein you consume. When you eat much fat to get enough calories needed by your body, you will be limiting fiber-rich foods such as vegetables, fruits, or legumes. These foods are some of the best sources of immune-boosting nutrients needed by your body to stay healthy. Therefore, when you limit these nutrients in your body, you increase your risk of getting chronic diseases such as diabetes, cancer, high blood pressure.

Studies show that diets that are high in fruits and vegetables can significantly reduce chronic diseases. The more you consume them, the better you are health-wise. When you restrict their consumption, you tend to decrease their beneficial impacts.

How to Reduce the Risk of Chronic Diseases When on Keto Diets

77

We'll say it again: drink lots of water. Eat lots of fruits and vegetables. You can also incorporate exercise into your keto diet to get the best results.

CHRONIC INFLAMMATION

Studies show that when you consume high fats needed for Ketosis, your cholesterol and lipoprotein structure could be significantly altered and will result in inflammation over a while. Inflammation occurs when the cells of your body use much energy to accomplish their normal functioning. Chronic inflammation is also one of the causes of heart diseases.

HOW TO MINIMIZE CHRONIC INFLAMMATION WHEN ON KETO

DIETS

You can control the problem of inflammation by eating solid fats and oils. Ensure you also include high fiber foods in your daily intake, like fruits and vegetables.

THE CHALLENGE OF WEIGHT CYCLING

When you restrict your eating diets for an extended period, you may end up gaining too much weight when not dieting, which you then go ahead and lose when on a diet. This process of alternating between weight gain and weight loss is what is referred to as weight cycling. Weight cycling can increase the risk of getting chronic diseases.

HOW TO CONTROL WEIGHT CYCLING

78

You can control weight cycling by shortening the intervals between dieting and the days you are on free diets. You should gradually increase the amount of food you consume during your free diet days so that your body can have enough time to adjust to the changes in your program.

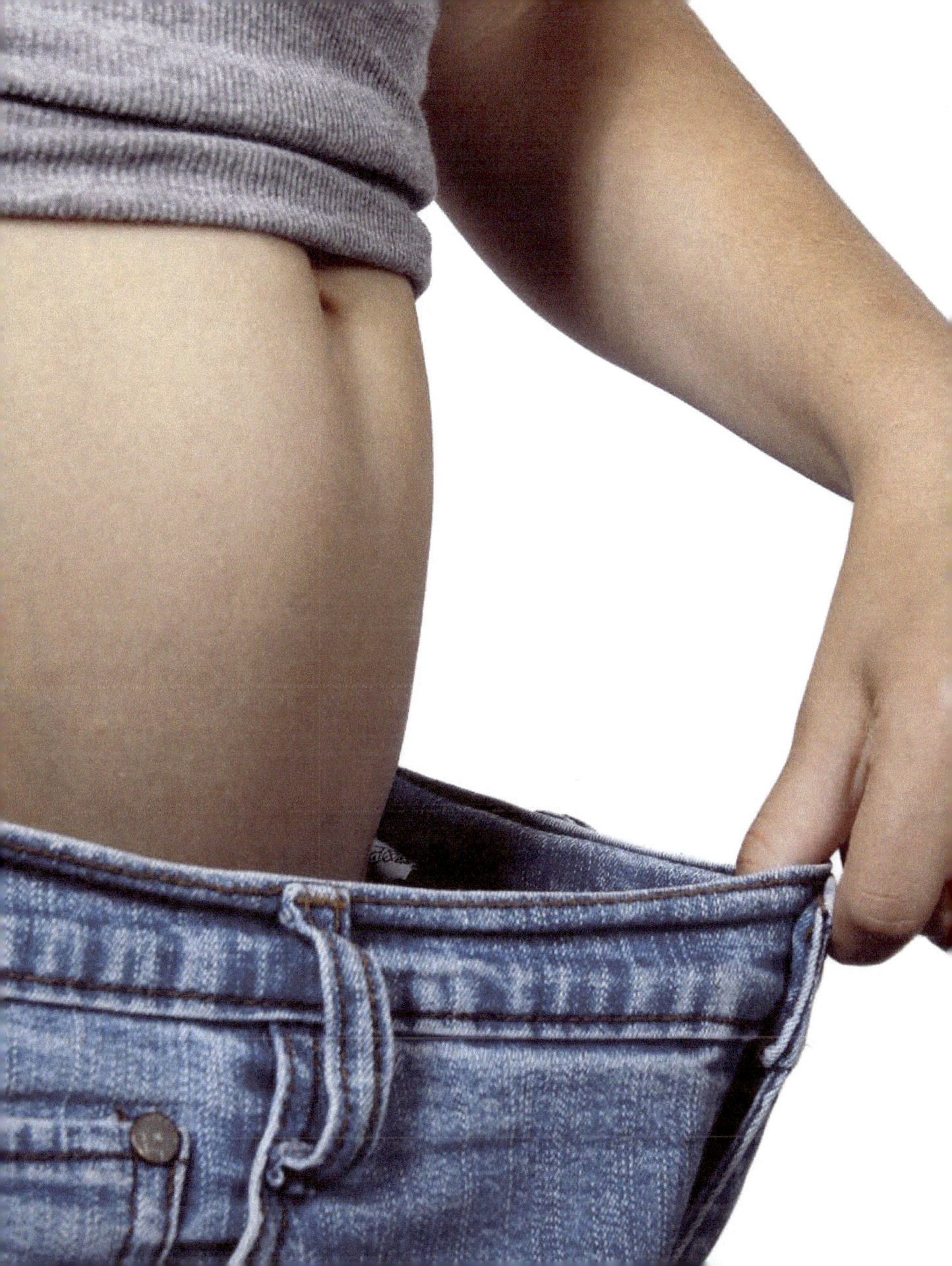

80

Chapter 10

Keto Diet and Intermittent Fasting

As we sail past 50, we will, in general, look out for things that will improve our experience in age, from serums and enhancements to diets, medications, and conventions. The items available are perpetual, however incidentally, perhaps the best thing you can accomplish for your maturing body doesn't include purchasing or getting tied up with anything.

You may have known about irregular fasting, which includes reasonable, exchanging times of eating and not eating, otherwise known as fasting. The exploration is entirely evident that intermittent fasting is gainful from numerous points of view, and this might be particularly valid for more seasoned grown-ups. The following are five advantages of intermittent fasting, alongside how to do it:

IT HELPS FIX CELLULAR FORMS IN YOUR BODY

The cellular part is not all bad as we age; however, fasting has been appeared to prompt your body's cell fix forms, improve hormone work, and even improves the capacity of qualities identified with sickness security and life span.

IT ADVANCES WEIGHT REDUCTION PARTICULARLY GUT FAT

Gut fat means that instinctive fat, which lies somewhere inside the stomach cavity, encompassing your organs and causing diseases. Losing gut fat is intense, particularly as we age, however as per an ongoing writing survey, discontinuous fasting can prompt loss from four to seven percent of your abdomen outline.

81

IT HELPS LESSENS AGGRAVATION AND OXIDATIVE PRESSURE

Irritation and oxidative pressure are significant supporters of ailment as we age, and they add to the unmistakable indications of maturing. This fasting decreases markers of oxidative pressure and irritation in overweight grown-ups.

IT MAY HELP PREVENT ALZHEIMER'S DISEASE

A massive collection of research shows that irregular fasting is useful for the mind, advancing the development of new nerve cells, shielding against cerebrum harm coming about because of stroke, and expanding levels of a hormone called brain determined neurotrophic factor or BDNF.

IT MAY EXTEND YOUR LIFE

82

A scope of ongoing examinations has additionally discovered that irregular fasting broadened the member's life expectancy. One examination found that rodents fasting each other day lived 83 percent longer than non-fasting rodents. Moreover, the maturing pace was eased back in the fasting rodents, and their body weight and development rates were decreased.

A TYPICAL SCHEDULE FOR THE 16/8 METHOD

Intermittent fasting is an eating plan on which you abandon nourishment for a specific measure of time. Furthermore, given the vast number of advantages (think weight reduction, glucose control, and even life span), it may not be a problem of whether you should attempt intermittent fasting yet, instead which kind of irregular fasting to attempt. If you are a freshman to fasting, you likely need to begin with 16:8; because of its implicit adaptability and simplicity to follow.

HOW THE 16/8 FASTING PLAN FUNCTIONS

The 16:8 fasting plan is an eating plan in which you embark on a fast for 16 hours every day then eat during an eight-hour window. This eating plan accompanies all the advantages of other fasting plans; besides, late research finds that it might bring down circulatory strain. Maybe far better, you pick the eating window.

If you know you're not strong enough to make no breakfast, space your nutriment prior in the day, about 8 a.m. to 4 p.m. On the off chance that you minded toward an early supper, eat in the day (11 a.m. to 6 p.m.). In case you're somebody who routinely goes out with companions for late suppers, plan your eating hours after the fact in the day will be 1 p.m. to 9 p.m.

83

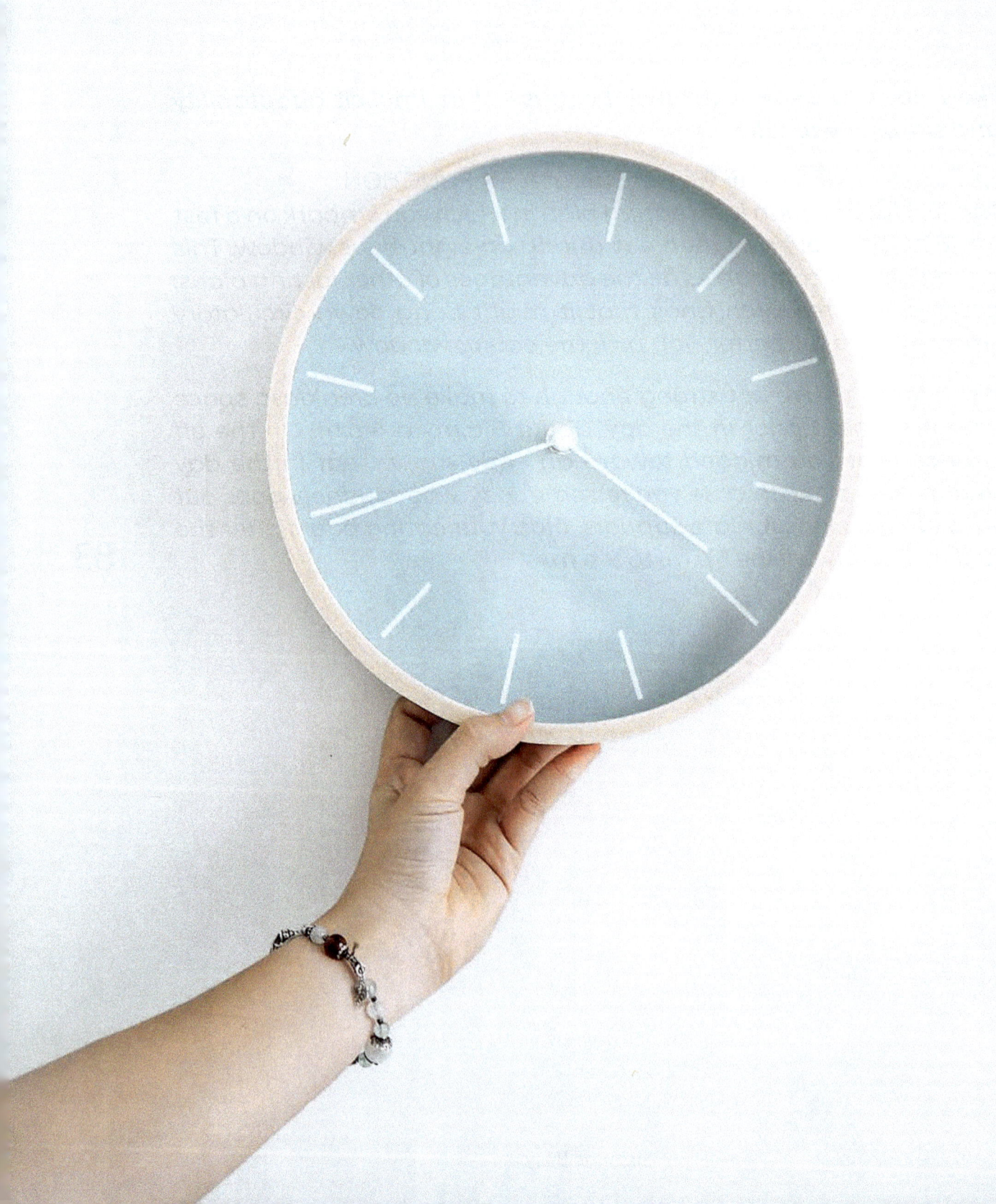

Chapter 11

The Importance of Exercising for Seniors and the Myths About

Exercising offers a plethora of benefits to all, regardless of your age! Healthy movement results in improved flexibility and stronger bones, which is quite important for older folks. You see, as you age, your body's muscle mass starts to decrease. As we enter our forties, adults begin to lose three to five percent of muscle mass as they enter each new decade.

However, we do realize how the thought of exercising regularly at an older age can seem like a challenge, especially if you're feeling let down with frequent aches and pains. But in many ways, the benefits of exercising outweigh the potential risks. Let's dive into why exercising is such an essential activity for seniors.

BENEFITS AND MYTHS OF EXERCISING FOR SENIORS

85

Now, while you may be having thoughts about exercising, here are a couple of benefits that you can't ignore:

PREVENTS DISEASES

Regular physical activity has been known to reduce the risks of diseases such as diabetes and heart disease. This is mainly because exercise strengthens overall immune functioning, which is particularly beneficial for seniors who are often immunocompromised. So even if you can't hit the gym, some form of light exercise can play an integral role in disease management.

HELPS INCREASE SOCIAL TIES AND PREVENTS ISOLATION

Aging can be a daunting process, but it becomes fun when you're surrounded by a community. Opting for yoga or fitness classes not only makes exercising more fun, but it also helps you strengthen social ties with other older adults in your neighborhood. This can help ward off the occasional loneliness that one is likely to feel at old age. Plus, this will help you stay committed to your goals and lead a healthier lifestyle.

IMPROVES COGNITIVE FUNCTION

Regular exercise can also improve fine motor skills that boost cognitive function. Several studies have shown how exercising can regularly reduce the risk of dementia.

Unfortunately, older folks have a higher risk of falling, which can lead to severe injuries. This can also drastically reduce your chances of leading an independent life as you grow older. As seniors take much longer to recover from injuries and falls, it is important to exercise to improve balance add mobility.

MYTHS

There are some myths associated with exercising for seniors. Let's debunk those misconceptions today:

Myth 1. I'm going to grow older; what's the point of exercising: Now, you might be thinking, "why should I exercise when moving around is likely to get difficult as I grow older?" Now here's the thing physical activity improves balance and helps you stay independent much longer. If you start exercising in your fifties, you are likely to have a better time moving around in your seventies, so start now.

86

Myth 2. I won't be great at exercising because I'm old: First off, you're never too old to exercise! So while strength and muscle mass tend to decline with age, that doesn't mean you can't partake in any form of physical activity. In fact, it's time you set healthier goals for yourself and improve your health. After all, isn't what this keto journey's all about? The key to exercising is finding activities that are suitable for you.

Living a sedentary lifestyle won't do you any good and will take a toll on your body.

Myth 3. I'll Be at a greater risk of falling down: If you're not careful, you will fall down regardless of your age. Regular physical activity builds stamina and strength. In many ways, exercising can help improve balance, reducing the risks of falling.

Myth 4. I'm not athletic I probably am not fit enough to exercise: Here's some news for you, our bodies are actually quite adjustable. So if you've suddenly decided to live a healthier lifestyle, nothing should stop you. So even if you're not athletic, that's perfectly fine; your body can still adjust to your new routine. Start with gentle activities such as brisk walking and then start building up from there.

Myth 5. I have a disability and can't exercise: People who are specially-abled or are chair-bound may find exercising challenging, but that doesn't mean you can't be part of the fan. Take up chair yoga or lift light weights. There are tons of simple exercises that can

87

help you improve the range of motion and flexibility. Speak to your doctor, and hopefully should have some great tips for you to follow.

SIMPLE EXERCISES FOR SENIORS

Here is a list of simple exercises that people in their fifties and beyond can enjoy:

LIGHT WEIGHT TRAINING

You can start off with a little weight training to retain bone density and build muscle mass. If you're more interested in doing home exercises than joining the gym, invest in 2-pound weights, and perform arm raises and shoulder presses.

88

Ideally, we recommend that you join a fitness center or gym where you can meet like-minded folks. You can also get yourself a personal trainer who can recommend customized workouts for you. Either way, remember to take it slow at first as you don't want to exert yourself too much.

WALKING

If lifting weights isn't for you, good old-fashioned walking should also work. Consider taking a nice walk around your neighborhood or go to a park nearby. You'll be able to make some friends and enjoy the weather while you're at it too.

In case you'd rather workout at home, strap on a pedometer, and get going around the house. You'll be able to get more out of this workout if you move your arms and lift your knees as you take each step.

AEROBICS

Joining an aerobics class can significantly help you keep your muscles strong whilst maintaining mobility. This will not only improve balance but will reduce the risk of falls, thus drastically improving the overall quality of your life as you grow older.

Many studies have also indicated how aerobic exercises can protect memory and sharpen your mind and improving cognitive function among older adults. If you're not comfortable joining a class, you'll find plenty of videos online. Aerobic exercises have also been known to get the heart pumping, improving cardiovascular help.

SWIMMING

Do you find regular exercise too boring? Swimming is a fun, impact-free exercise that can get you through the day. It's almost pain-free and won't trouble your aging joints. Swimming offers resistance training and will help you get back up to your feet again.

Here's how it works: the water offers gentle resistance while giving you a cardiovascular workout too. This also builds muscle capacity and helps you build strength too.

YOGA

What's no to love about yoga? It's relaxing, it's healthy, and you can enjoy it with a group. Yoga does an excellent job improving flexibility in your joints. It allows seniors to remain limber and maintain their sense of balance. If you have trouble moving about or stretching, then you can try chair yoga.

Some classic yoga poses that you might want to try out include seated forward bend, downward-facing dog, and warrior.

SQUATS

When you're working on an exercise program, you shouldn't skip the idea of strength training. Squats happen to be an excellent way to strengthen the muscles of your lower body. Doing squats is relatively easy, and you won't need any sort of equipment except for maybe a chair to support yourself. However, if you have trouble with balance, we suggest you skip this exercise and opt for something much simpler.

SIT-UPS

Sit-ups are a great way to strengthen your core muscles, improve back pain problems, and balance. Performing simple sit-ups should do the job. All you have to do is lie down on your back and keep your knees bent at an angle. Now place your hands behind your head and then gently try to lift your head. You should feel the sensation in your core muscles.

90

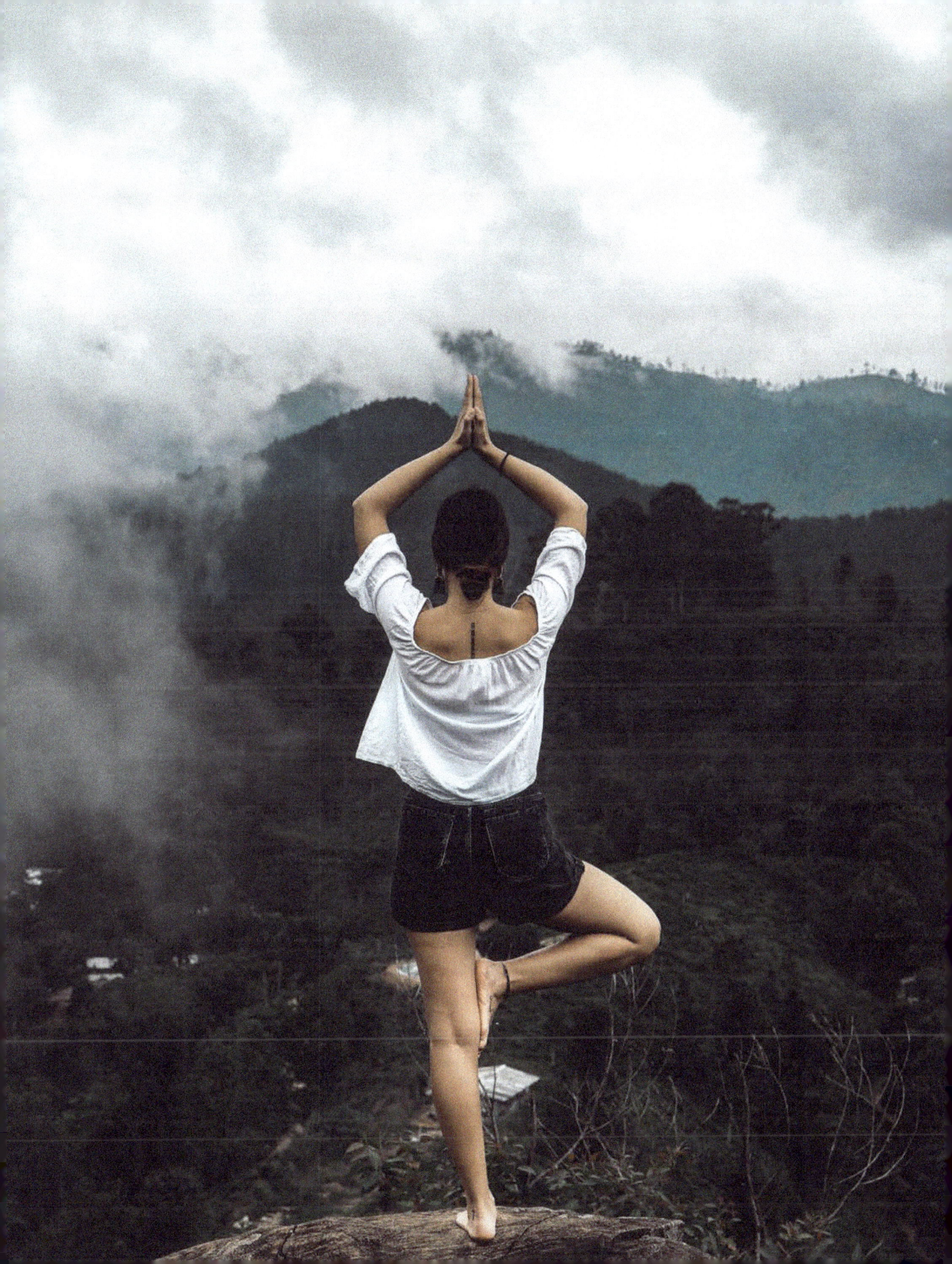

92

Chapter 12

Keto Food List

Now, let's dive straight into the things that actually matter. Let's discover all about food, what to eat, and what to say goodbye to. I will provide you with some great tips to help you with your selection, to ensure that you always end up with the finest quality and enjoy every ounce of the scrumptious recipes you will create using these food items.

I will provide you with some nutritional facts, and we will eventually look into what exactly macros and calories are and how we can keep track of all that is important.

THE RICHNESS WITHIN KETO

Food. Without it, we would be doomed. Keto, obviously, would fare no better either. But the presence of all the enormous types and kinds of food isn't exactly helping the case either. For starters, we are not out to grab everything that packs a punch. We are more interested in food items that help our case and provide us with the specific nutrients we are seeking.

93

Remember, keto is a high-fat and low-carb diet. When I say "low carb," I do really mean low; 20-50 grams of it in a day. That is quite a challenge for some.

It is important to remember the above and follow the guidelines set in place. With that said, let's move further ahead and see what kind of food items we can use.

THE GOOD

Let me list down some of the healthiest keto foods that you can get your hands on today from your local market. These do not cost much and add quite a bit of value and taste to your meal.

SEAFOOD

Keto diet loves seafood, and that is as simple as that. Fish like salmon are packed with vitamin B and selenium, along with potassium too. The beauty behind it is that these are extremely low in carbs, so low that these are almost free of carbs in most cases.

I did say almost, which is why it is best to keep track of your carb intake.

When it comes to shellfish, the amount of carb varies. If you love crab or have a thing for shrimp, rejoice! These contain no carbs. For others, you may wish to double-check.

Now, since our daily limit for carbs consumption is rather tight, you may wish to start paying attention to the number of carbs some of the shellfish have. A count for some popular ones is shown here (100 grams or 3.5 ounces):

- *Mussels: 7 grams*

- *Oysters: 4 grams*

- *Clams: 5 grams*

- *Octopus: 4 grams*

94

- *Squid: 3 grams*

The good news for those who love other fish like mackerel or sardines, these two, along with salmon, are extremely rich in omega-3 fats. It has been shown in various studies that this helps keep your insulin levels low. Fish intake also improves your mental health, so there is just so much goodness on offer here.

Twice a week is a good frequency, something for you to remember.

LOW CARB VEGGIES

They exist! They most certainly do and have been with us for a very long time. The issue was that we never paid much attention to these—time to find out which ones made it into the world of keto.

Pretty much most non-starchy veggies are quite low in terms of calories. They are significantly low in carbs as well, but they do come with higher values when it comes to other nutrients. That would also include vitamin C, in case you were looking for it.

95

The problem with vegetables and plants is that they come with fiber, and our body doesn't exactly digest that, and that causes a bit of a miscalculation. To get the right values, try and seek out net carb count, which is essentially fiber deducted from the total carbs.

"So, it's okay to consume potatoes, then?" Not quite. You see, potatoes, yams, and beets contain starch, and just a single serving of these is enough to send your carbohydrate count through the roof for the day. Keep a very strict check on potatoes as these are

especially hard to avoid.

Vegetables also contain antioxidants that help by protecting us against free radicals that cause damage to our bodies. Broccoli, kale, and cauliflower also play a significant part in keeping heart issues and cancer at bay—all the more reasons for you to include veggies.

CHEESE

Yes, please! Without cheese, we would be left in a world that is just tasteless in most cases. The cheese is delicious and nutritious as well. The best part is that all types of cheese are low in carbs and high in fats. It's like they were created with keto in mind, or maybe the entire keto diet was created by someone who preferred cheese. Either way, it's a win-win for us all.

96

While cheese is high in saturated fats, there are no such studies to show that it causes an increased risk of cardiac diseases, and that is good news for everyone.

Contrary to popular belief, cheese contains what are called conjugated linoleic acid. In simple English, it is a fat that helps with fat loss, which is odd but nonetheless helpful.

Since we are 50 or more in age, cheese does help us in reducing the loss of muscles, which is only natural at this age.

AVOCADO

Without a doubt, the best ingredient of the lot. Use it on its own or mix it with various food items, and you always get that great sensation, a punch of great taste, and great nutritional values.

For every 100 grams of avocados, roughly around one-half of a medium-sized avocado, you only get nine grams of carbs. If that raised some curiosity, here's another fact: seven of those grams are fiber. That means you are only consuming two grams of carbs. That is just phenomenal.

They help you improve your cholesterol levels; they hold a high dose of some important vitamins and minerals, and the higher potassium makes everything a little easier during the transition to keto.

MEAT AND POULTRY

Of course, meals are never considered complete without meat and poultry. The good news is that you have a diverse range of these available as good keto food. The only catch is that you must buy your meat and poultry fresh.

97

Fresh meat and poultry are free from carbs and contain high vitamin B counts. Potassium, zinc, and selenium are loaded too, and that further helps our goal.

However, the main reason we go for this is protein. Needless to say, these are some of the finest sources of proteins that help us in preserving our muscle mass throughout the low carb diet.

When choosing your meat, opt for grass-fed meat. This option is *safe and comes with all the goodness we seek.*

EGGS

Cheap, easy to make, and delicious when cooked right. Eggs are one of the most versatile foods on the face of the earth.

Just to give you an idea of how great these are, one large egg only holds less than one gram of carbs and six grams of protein. That, then, makes eggs the ideal food for anyone following the ketogenic diet.

Studies have shown that eggs trigger the release of hormones, which give us a feeling of fullness while keeping our blood sugar levels intact. When consuming eggs, ensure you eat the complete egg to get the most nutrients from the yolk as well.

98

Now I know, some may be quick to point out that yolks contain high cholesterol, but the fact is that these do not raise cholesterol levels in most people. However, to make things easier, consult your doctor first to find out if you can consume eggs regularly.

NUTS AND SEEDS

No talk about protein is ever complete without the mention of nuts and seeds. Those who are comfortable consuming these are in for a treat.

To provide you with an idea of how much these offers, here is a list of some common nuts and seeds and their carb values (28 grams or 1 ounce):

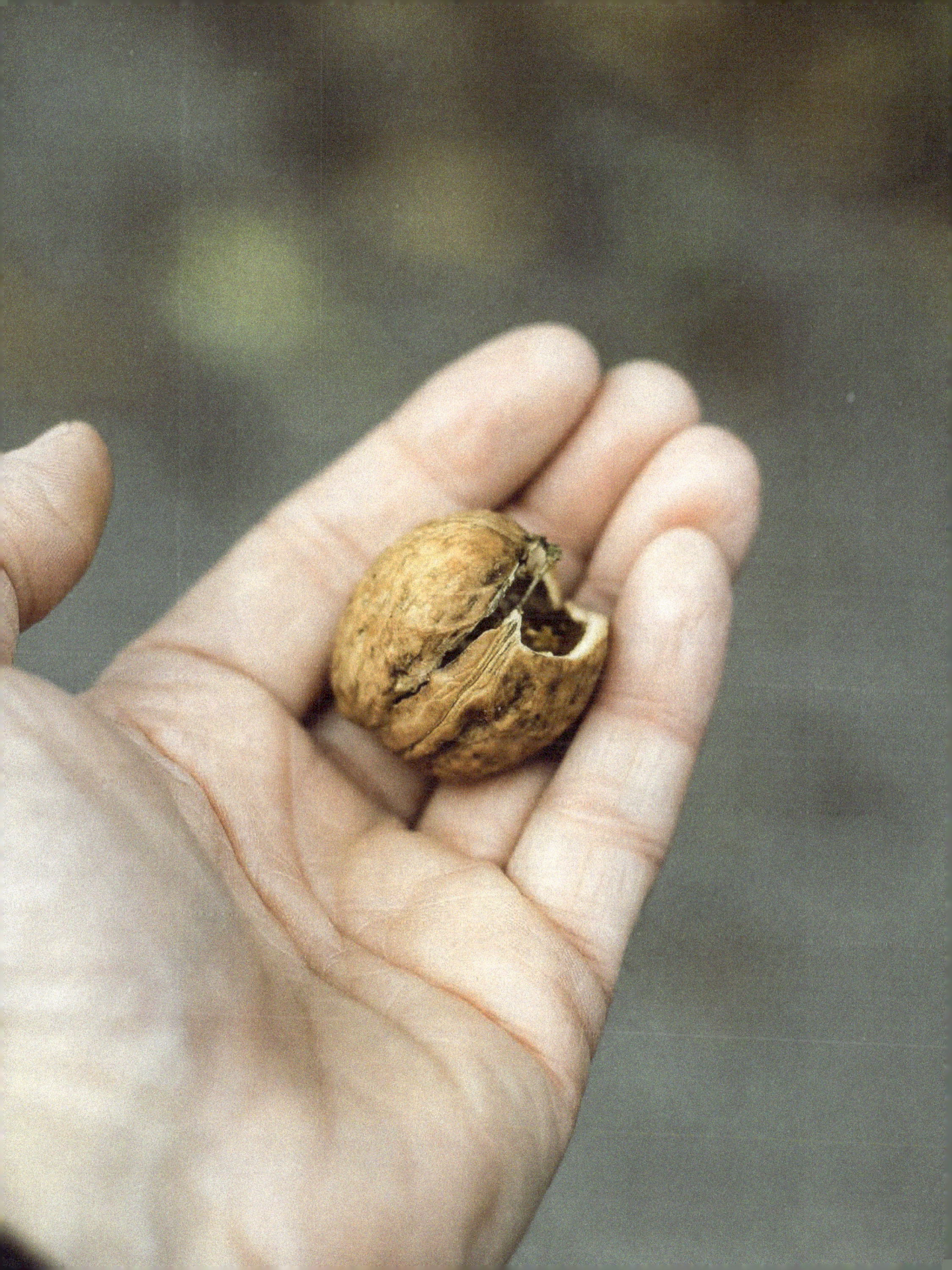

- *Almonds - 3 grams*

- *Brazil nuts - 1 gram*

- *Cashews - 8 grams*

- *Chia Seeds - 1 gram*

- *Flaxseeds - 0 grams*

- *Macadamia nuts - 2 grams*

- *Pecans - 1 gram*

- *Pistachios - 5 grams*

- *Pumpkin Seeds - 4 grams*

- *Sesame seeds - 3 grams*

- *Walnuts - 2 grams*

OTHER FOOD ITEMS

Frankly, this list continues to grow almost every year. However, to give you a quick view of what you can expect to eat, here are some other food items included and considered genuinely good within the keto circle.

- *Coconut Oil*

- *Olive Oil*

100

- *Plain Greek Yogurt*

- *Cottage Cheese*

- *Berries*

- *Butter and Cream*

- *Shirataki Noodles*

- *Olives*

- *Unsweetened Coffee*

- *Unsweetened Tea*

- *Dark Chocolate*

- *Cocoa Powder*

101

Interestingly enough, that pretty much covers almost everything that one may require. However, it is time to move on to the things you should avoid at all costs when observing the keto diet.

The Bad and the Ugly

I will not dwindle on about how these things can be bad or what they can do to you in much detail. However, I will let you know that most of these are already rich in carbs, which automatically renders them ineligible to be made a part of your keto diet.

BREAD AND GRAINS

No matter what form bread takes, they still pack a lot of carbs. The same applies to whole-grain as well because they are made from refined flour. So, if you want to eat bread, it is best to make keto variants at home instead.

Grains such as rice, wheat, and oats pack a lot of carbs. So, limit or avoid that as well.

FRUITS

Fruits are healthy for you. The problem is that some of those foods pack quite a lot of carbs, such as banana, raisins, dates, mango, and pear. As a general rule, avoid sweet and dried fruits.

VEGETABLES

Vegetables are just as healthy for your body. For one, they make you feel full for longer, so they help suppress your appetite. But that also means you need to avoid or limit vegetables that are high in starch because they have more carbs than fiber. That includes corn, potato, sweet potato, and beets.

PASTA

As with any other convenient food, pasta is rich in carbs. So, spaghetti or any different types of pasta are not recommended when you are on your keto diet.

CEREAL

Cereal is also a considerable offender because sugary breakfast cereals pack a lot of carbs. That also applies to "healthy cereals." Just because they use other words to describe their product does not

102

mean that you should believe them. That also applies to oatmeal, whole-grain cereals, etc.

BEER

In reality, you can drink most alcoholic beverages in moderation without fear. Beer is an exception to this rule because it packs a lot of carbs. Carbs in beers or other liquid are considered liquid carbs, and they are even more dangerous than substantial carbs.

SWEETENED YOGURT

Yogurt is very healthy because it is tasty and does not have that many carbs. The problem comes when you consume yogurt variants rich in carbs such as fruit-flavored, low-fat, sweetened, or nonfat yogurt. A single serving of sweetened yogurt contains as many carbs as a single serving of dessert.

103

JUICE

Fruit juices are perhaps the worst beverage you can put into your system when you are on a keto diet. Another problem is that the brain does not process liquid carbs the same way as stable carbs. Substantial carbs can help suppress appetite, but liquid carbs will only put your need into overdrive.

LOW-FAT AND FAT-FREE SALAD DRESSINGS

If you have to buy salads, keep in mind that commercial sauces pack more carbs than you think, especially the fat-free and low-fat variants.

Beans and Legumes

These are also very nutritious as they are rich in fiber. However, they are also rich in carbs. You may enjoy a small amount of them when you are on your keto diet, but don't exceed your carb limit.

SUGAR

We mean sugar in any form, including honey. Foods that contain lots of sugar, such as cookies, candies, and cake, are forbidden on a keto diet or any other form of diet that is designed to lose weight. When you are on a keto diet, you need to keep in mind that your diet consists of food that is rich in fiber and nutritious. So, sugar is out of the question.

CHIPS AND CRACKERS

These two are some of the most popular snacks. Some people did not realize that one packet of chips contains several servings and should not be all eaten in one go. The carbs can add up very quickly if you do not watch what you eat.

104

MILK

Milk also contains a lot of carbs on its own. Therefore, avoid it if you can even though milk is a good source of many nutrients such as calcium, potassium, and other B vitamins.

GLUTEN-FREE BAKED GOODS

Gluten-free diets are trendy nowadays, but what many people don't seem to realize is that they pack quite a lot of carbs. That includes gluten-free bread, muffins, and other baked products. In reality, they contain even more carbs than their glutenous variant.

Chapter 13

30-Day Keto Diet Weight Loss Meal Plan

This contains a 30-day meal plan for Keto Diet to help you eat the right amount of food and keep track of daily intake. Also, to avoid the food you should not eat in the Keto diet. The meal plan will help you save a lot of time since your meal is already planned and avoids wasting food. Furthermore, the meal plan saves you a lot of money and refrain you from eating outside. The meal plan provides you with nutritionally well-balanced meals throughout the week. Meals from breakfast, lunch, dinner, and snack are provided for your convenience.

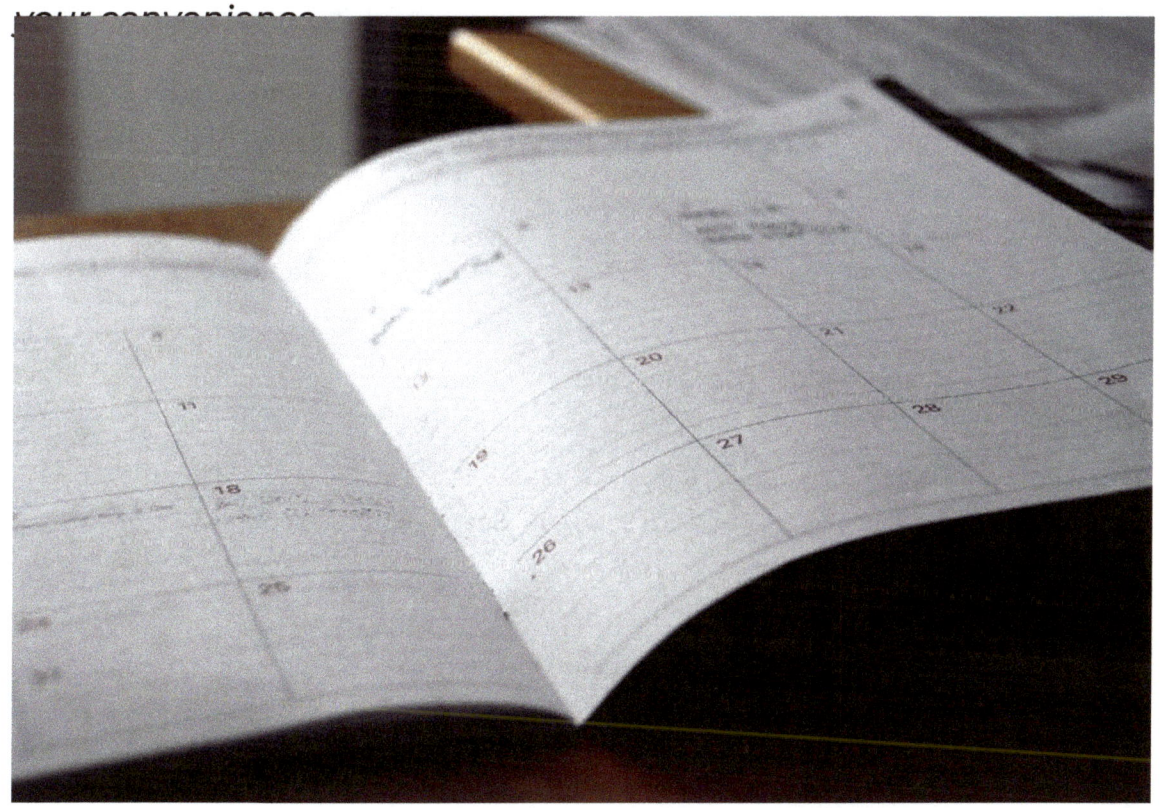

105

Day	Breakfast	Lunch	Dinner	Snack
1	Bacon Cheeseburger Waffles	Green Beans Salad	Korma Curry	Keto Cheesecakes
2	Keto Breakfast Cheesecake	Apple Salad	Zucchini Bars	Keto Brownies
3	Egg-Crust Pizza	Asian Salad	Mushroom Soup	Raspberry and Coconut
4	Breakfast Roll-Ups	Octopus Salad	Stuffed Portobello Mushrooms	Chocolate Pudding Delight
5	Basic Opie Rolls	Shrimp Salad	Lettuce Salad	Peanut Butter Fudge
6	Almond Coconut Egg Wraps	Lamb Salad	Onion Soup	Cinnamon Streusel Egg Loaf
7	Bacon & Avocado Omelet	Coconut Soup	Asparagus Salad	Snickerdoodle Muffins
8	Bacon & Cheese Frittata	Broccoli Soup	Beef with Cabbage Noodles	Yogurt and Strawberry Bowl
9	Bacon & Egg Breakfast Muffins	Simple Tomato Soup	Roast Beef and Mozzarella Plate	Sweet Cinnamon Muffin

106

10	Bacon Hash	Green Soup	Beef and Broccoli	Nutty Muffins
11	Bagels With Cheese	Sausage and Peppers Soup	Garlic Herb Beef Roast	Pumpkin and Cream Cheese Cup
12	Baked Apples	Avocado Soup	Sprouts Stir-fry with Kale, Broccoli, and Beef	Berries in Yogurt Cream
13	Baked Eggs In The Avocado	Avocado and Bacon Soup	Beef and Vegetable Skillet	Pumpkin Pie Mug Cake
14	Banana Pancakes	Roasted Bell Peppers Soup	Beef, Pepper and Green Beans Stir-fry	Chocolate and Strawberry Crepe
15	Breakfast Skillet	Spicy Bacon Soup	Cheesy Meatloaf	Blackberry and Coconut Flour Cupcake
16	Brunch BLT Wrap	Taco Stuffed Avocados	Roast Beef and Vegetable Plate	Keto Cheesecakes
17	Korma Curry	Buffalo Shrimp Lettuce Wraps	Breakfast Roll-Ups	Keto Brownies
18	Zucchini Bars	Keto Bacon Sushi	Basic Opie Rolls	Raspberry and Coconut

107

108

19	Mushroom Soup	Keto Burger Fat Bombs	Almond Coconut Egg Wraps	Chocolate Pudding Delight
20	Stuffed Portobello Mushrooms	Caprese Zoodles	Bacon & Avocado Omelet	Peanut Butter Fudge
21	Lettuce Salad	Zucchini Sushi	Bacon & Cheese Frittata	Cinnamon Streusel Egg Loaf
22	Onion Soup	Asian Chicken Lettuce Wraps	Bacon & Egg Breakfast Muffins	Snickerdoodle Muffins
23	Asparagus Salad	Prosciutto and Mozzarella Bomb	Bacon Hash	Yogurt and Strawberry Bowl
24	Beef with Cabbage Noodles	Ketofied Chick-Fil-A-style Chicken	Bagels with Cheese	Sweet Cinnamon Muffin
25	Roast Beef and Mozzarella Plate	Cheeseburger Tomatoes	Baked Apples	Nutty Muffins
26	Beef and Broccoli	Green Beans Salad	Baked Eggs In The Avocado	Pumpkin and Cream Cheese Cup
27	Garlic Herb Beef Roast	Apple Salad	Banana Pancakes	Berries in Yogurt Cream

28	Sprouts Stir-fry with Kale, Broccoli, and Beef	Asian Salad	Breakfast Skillet	Pumpkin Pie Mug Cake
29	Beef and Vegetable Skillet	Octopus Salad	Breakfast Roll-Ups	Chocolate and Strawberry Crepe
30	Beef, Pepper and Green Beans Stir-fry	Shrimp Salad	Basic Opie Rolls	Blackberry and Coconut Flour Cupcake

109

110

Conclusion

Your dedication to improve your health and lose weight is phenomenal since you have been able to reach the end of this book. It is not an easy process to lose weight; if you are able to maintain the guidelines you have learned in this book and stay motivated; your life will change in ways that you cannot imagine. You are on the right track to achieve both mental and physical health. Even though adjusting to eating a healthy diet after being accustomed to eating a lot of convenience foods is a challenge, you will feel the difference in energy levels that you will experience. You will look good and be safe from many of the common nutrition-related diseases and conditions, and on top of all of that, your quality of life will improve greatly.

We are all different; thus, you should take time to really understand what a weight loss program involves and try out the program gradually. If you nose dive into a weight loss program is not advisable since it may not be for you. No regiment works perfectly for everyone; thus, you should select a plan and modify it in a way that suits you. There are many weight loss programs with mind-blowing results, but they may be too hard to follow or just unsafe to practice.

You work out intensity, duration, your resting period are all factors that should be considered. It best works when it is a constant in your daily activity, and as it is not a permanent change of your physical and psychological condition.

111

In order to get the maximum weight loss experience, you should listen to your body. This does not mean that you should eat any time you feel hungry; it means that you should listen to how it responds to your diet and fasting regiment because the body system determines the time for you to eat, time for you to exercise, and even how many calories you take in. Thus you will be in full control of your weight loss once you are in control of your diet and fasting program.

You should know that even though the ketogenic diet is about carbohydrate restriction, do not excessively restrict them; you should make sure you eat enough. If you restrict calories too much, you will be moody, and it can even stop your fat loss process. You should also vary your food choices so that you make sure that you are getting the nutrients you need so as to maintain your health.

112

In fact, getting all the nutrients that you require from a ketogenic diet is possible. Unfortunately for some, this is not possible. If you do not feel okay, you should go and see a doctor so as to determine if you have any nutritional deficiencies. He/she will able to recommend supplements for you from that information.

For health reasons, weight loss should be a slow process. Losing 2 pounds a day is okay, but anything more than that is a lot. Engage in your day-to-day operations while fasting as this is a time-flying route. Good luck with your keto diet journey!